WEE TIPS, ON KNEES & HIPS

Information on Knee & Hip Implants and More

Shahrzad Shariatpanahi, BSc, MSc

Biomedical Engineer & STEM Ambassador

Copyright © 2020 Shahrzad Shariatpanahi

All rights reserved

No part of this book may be reproduced, stored in a retrieval system, or transmitted in any form or by any means, electronic, mechanical, photocopying, recording, or otherwise, without express written permission of the author and the publisher.

ISBN: 9798648485570

Dedicated to the loving memory of my late grandfathers, Seifollah & Ziauddin.

Shahrzad, October 2023

I am dedicating this book to

MY AMAZING PARENTS

Who consistently showed me unwavering love, believed in me, and spurred me on to reach my fullest potential.

MY REMARKABLE HUSBAND

Who has been the most encouraging and supportive presence in my life, and I am immensely grateful.

MY BRILLIANT SISTER

Her exceptional intelligence and determined spirit serve as a constant source of inspiration.

Contents

List of figures vi

Preface xix

Introduction xxv

Disclaimer xxviii

Chapter 1 - A Historical Survey of Joint Replacement **1**

A concise history of joint diseases, p.2; historical evidence of joint disease in Britain, p.6; historical development of surgical principles, p.10; setting and fixing fractures, p.12; alignment and stability, p.12; orthopaedic surgery advancements, p.17; total hip replacement (THR), p.17; total knee replacement (TKR), p.22; groundbreaking advancements in joint surgery, p.26; total joint replacement or arthroplasty, p.35; joint replacement in contemporary times, p.52; bilateral joint arthroplasty, p.74.

Chapter 2 - The Hip Joint   81

An introduction to the hip joint, p.82; anatomical planes and motion axes, p.83; anatomy and biomechanics of the hip joint, p.86; the pelvis, p.91; the femur, p.96; hip implants, p.98; femoral component or stem, p.104; stem material and surface finish, p.109; femoral head, p.114; head options, p.117, acetabular liner, p.123; liner material, p.124; head-liner combinations, p.126; liner locking or fixation designs, p.128; acetabular shell, P.132; variety of shapes and sizes, p.133; cup fixation options, p.134; acetabular component material and coating, p.136; primary vs. revision hip implants, p.137.

Chapter 3 - The Knee Joint**143**

An introduction to the knee joint, p.144; anatomy and biomechanics of the knee joint, p.147; knee implants, p.176; total knee replacement, p.177; femoral component, p.178; polyethylene insert, p.179; tibial component, tray or baseplate, p.180; patellar component, p.181; partial (unicompartmental) knee replacement, p.184; bicompartmental knee replacement, p.191; kneecap or patellofemoral arthroplasty, p.192; TKA implant design and materials, p.195; femoral component, p.196; tibial component, p.198; tibial insert design, p.201; the inferior surface of the insert (tibial locking), p.208; modular tibial tray or baseplate, p.211; primary vs. revision knee implants, p.213.

Chapter 4 - Joint Replacement Journey 221

Pre-operative preparation, p.222; physical preparation, p.224; home preparation, p.225; other preparations, p.226; preparing your post-op living environment, p.230; home safety checklist, p.231; the patient on the day of the surgery, p.234; medical team on the day of the surgery, p.241; post-op journey, p.244; a few more tips to consider, p.252; post-operative (after surgery) general instructions, p.259; revision THA/TKA, p.263; common reasons for revision, p.269.

Chapter 5 - Appendices   **275**

Glossary, p.276; gold/brass coloured components, p.292; BMI or body mass index, p.295; pre-surgery preparation checklist, p.300.

List of figures

Figure 1-1 Hunting woolly mammoth   3

Figure 1-2 Life in the 19th century   4

Figure 1-3 Life expectancy history from 1950 to 2020 (United Kingdom) ©2023 WolframAlpha 5

Figure 1-4 Left: early Romano-British adult female, right: remains of a Romano-British decapitation burial of a juvenile, accompanied by a lamb ©2013 WessexArch   7

Figure 1-5 Left: a healthy knee joint. Right: a knee joint affected by rheumatoid arthritis   9

Figure 1-6 Application of Thomas Splint - a common orthopaedic equipment in hospitals worldwide. First description by Hugh Owen Thomas published in 1875   11

Figure 1-7 An 18th century operating room 16

Figure 1-8 Sir John Charnley at Wrightington Hospital (by Evening Standard/Getty Images) 19

Figure 1-9 Professor Themistocles Gluck (by Prof. Munjed Al Muderis)   22

Figure 1-10 Left: John Insall, MD. Right: the Insall Burstein Posterior Stabilised I Knee prosthesis was designed to substitute for the posterior cruciate ligament (by Giles R. Scuderi, MD)   24

Figure 1-11 Professor Anthony White (by Chelsea and Westminster Hospital)   26

Figure 1-12 Biographical sketch: Themistocles Gluck (1853–1942) © SpringerLink   29

Figure 1-13 Judet acrylic femoral head (by Dr Prakash) 32

Figure 1-14 Left: an unhealthy & painful knee joint, right: a total knee joint replacement (by ADAM) 35

Figure 1-15 Hip prosthetic components engineered to mimic the natural movement and function of the joint as closely as possible (by Alila Medical Images/Alamy Stock Photo) 38

Figure 1-16 A normal, OA, and RA joint 43

Figure 1-17 OA vs RA 48

Figure 1-18 Joint replacement surgery 51

Figure 1-19 Top: life expectancy in 2020-2025, bottom: life expectancy in 1950-1955 53

Figure 1-20 First modern hip replacement (low friction prostheses) by Sir John Charnley   57

Figure 1-21 The mean BMI, from top to bottom: women in 1975 (22), men in 1975 (21.5), women in 2016 (25) & men in 2016 (24.5). Note the dotted line indicates average BMI in the UK ©2017 NCD Risk Factor Collaboration   65

Figure 1-22 Obesity prevalence in the UK between the years 1975 and 2016 separated by gender ©2017 NCD Risk Factor   68

Figure 1-23 An increase in the rate of primary total hip replacement operations   71

Figure 1-24 The activity scale for knee   73

Figure 1-25 Bilateral TKR and unilateral (left side) THR (by ChooChin / Getty Images)   76

Figure 2-1 Visualisation of the anatomical reference planes and axes 85

Figure 2-2 The hip joint provides the following movements: abduction, adduction, flexion, extension and internal and external rotation 86

Figure 2-3 Right hip joint 88

Figure 2-4 Possible hip movements 90

Figure 2-5 The pelvis bone, lateral (left) and medial (right) view 93

Figure 2-6 Keep essential items at reach 95

Figure 2-7 The angle of inclination's impact on the knee joint alignment 97

Figure 2-8 Left: hemiarthroplasty, right: total hip replacement 98

Figure 2-9 Monoblock (a), vs modular (b, c) hip system (by Irena Gotman) 99

Figure 2-10 Hemiarthroplasty 101

Figure 2-11 Metal-on-metal hip resurfacing system - "M-o-M" means that both the joint's ball and socket components are made of metal 103

Figure 2-12 The above poster published in 2003, courtesy of Annie Gallup, is the display of various designs of modular and mono-block THA femoral components 106

Figure 2-13 Two examples of femoral component designs (there are several other designs available on the market) 108

Figure 2-14 Common types of surface finish for femoral stems 110

Figure 2-15 U2 hip system, porous coating (left), HA coating (middle) and smooth surface finish (right) 112

Figure 2-16 Bone cement application in THA (by Vasilios Athans) 113

Figure 2-17 A retrieved modular femoral head made of Alumina ceramic 114

Figure 2-18 From left to right: stainless steel, Co-Cr, Alumina ceramic, Zirconia ceramic and Oxinium™ modular femoral heads 116

Figure 2-19 Femoral head options 118

Figure 2-20 Three designs for femoral heads: unipolar, bipolar, and dual mobility 120

Figure 2-21 Liners (a) HXL-UHMWPE, (b) Vitamin E-blended HXLUHMWPE (by Takahashi) 123

Figure 2-22 Metal stem head, liner & cup making a M-o-M bearing which is no longer on the market (By Gregory A. Tocks, D.O.) 125

Figure 2-23 Head-liner combination example 127

Figure 2-24 Liner fixation e.g., anti-rotation device (ARD) design & lipped/elevated design 129

Figure 2-25 Left: uncemented (ARD) design, right: cemented liner design (by Barrios) 131

Figure 2-26 Hemispherical vs elliptical shell 133

Figure 2-27 Left: a cementless (metal) acetabular shell, right: a cemented (polyethylene) acetabular cup (by D.S.Angadi) 134

Figure 2-28 Left: a primary total hip replacement, right: a revision total hip replacement. Note the difference in the size & shape of the parts 139

Figure 3-1 Right tibia superior 147

Figure 3-2 Knee joint anterolateral 148

Figure 3-3 Frontal plane deviations of the knee, top: normal, bottom: varus & valgus 150

Figure 3-4 "Genu varum"/"genu valgum" 154

Figure 3-5 Soft tissue surrounding knee 162

Figure 3-6 Knee bursae 165

Figure 3-7 Knee menisci 167

Figure 3-8 Ligaments (by Dr Gambardella) 171

Figure 3-9 Knee extension motion 175

Figure 3-10 Partial vs total knee system 176

Figure 3-11 Total knee femoral component 178

Figure 3-12 Total knee polyethylene component or tibial insert or plastic spacer 179

Figure 3-13 Total knee tibial tray 180

Figure 3-14 Some examples of TKA patellar component (by Oliver S. Schindler) 182

Figure 3-15 Unicompartmental knee implant 185

Figure 3-16 Illustration and X-ray image of medial compartment osteoarthritis of the knee (by Michael M. Alexiades, MD) 186

Figure 3-17 Preservation of healthy knee joint structures, including ligaments and bone, in the non-affected compartments 188

Figure 3-18 UKA & TKA posterior view 190

Figure 3-19 Bicompartmental knee 191

Figure 3-20 Patellofemoral alignment 193

Figure 3-21 The Episealer Implant 194

Figure 3-22 Total knee replacement comp. 197

Figure 3-23 Left: Anatomic Graduated Component (AGC), right: mono block tibial component 199

Figure 3-24 Anterior stabilised (A), and posterior stabilised (B) tibial insert (by Yong In, MD) 201

Figure 3-25 Polyethylene insert types 202

Figure 3-26 Two mobile bearing designs 207

Figure 3-27 Left: Fixed-bearing TKR, right: mobile-bearing or rotating platform (RP) TKR 209

Figure 3-28 Two TKR tibial tray designs, fixed bearing & rotating platform 211

Figure 3-29 Top & bottom view of 4 separate tibial components (Nexgen, Attune, Triathlon, PFC) & corresponding PE inserts (by R.Bhalekar) 212

Figure 3-30 Left: primary total knee replacement, right: revision TKR 214

Figure 3-31 Four degrees of bone loss in revision total knee arthroplasty 219

Figure 4-1 Better your lifestyle (Dr. Sangeeta) 223

Figure 4-2 A cluttered living area makes it hard to move with a walking frame 225

Figure 4-3 *No paint on nails during surgery* 229

Figure 4-4 Mark the correct joint 235

Figure 4-5 Overnight Hospital Bag by Hugbag 236

Figure 4-6 Recovering from joint replacement is like a marathon, not a sprint, requiring time and dedication 251

Figure 4-7 Examples of the DIY little bag, caddy and water bottle holder for walking aids (scan the corresponding QR codes to access each website/tutorial) 253

Figure 4-8 Top left: picking up or reaching assist tool, top right: pants lift & slip aid, bottom: sock aid device. All available to purchase online 258

Figure 4-9 Mobility aids 260

Figure 4-10 Top left: aseptic loosening of the stem, right: adverse tissue reaction to debris, bottom left: subluxation/partial dislocation, right: dislocation of the right hip head 268

Figure 4-11 Top reasons for revision THR 272

Figure 4-12 Top reasons for revision TKR 273

Preface

I'm a Biomedical Engineer, and my journey into the world of orthopaedic implants began in 2009. It all started with my academic studies, and as I pursued my career, I continued to delve into this field. Along the way, I've acquired knowledge about various aspects of joint replacement including the implants, their designs, the materials used in manufacturing these implants, and the factors that can lead to them not working as intended. I've also kept up with the latest research worldwide to stay informed about the most up-to-date developments in all orthopaedic implants including hip and knee replacements.

I am fascinated to learn more about people who have undergone hip or knee replacement, their experiences, emotions, and what they hope for. I want to grasp how getting a new joint would impact a person's daily life, mental well-being, social interactions, and relationships. In order to do this, I explore information online and read about the experiences of patients. I also participate in events and gatherings; online forums and social media groups dedicated to hip and knee replacements and engage with participants.

I suggest that you also consider doing this, as it will enable you to connect with a group of individuals who have shared a similar experience. Hopefully, this will reassure you that you're not alone on your joint replacement journey. Many individuals are going through what you're experiencing, some recovering swiftly and maybe a few facing post-surgery challenges.

Throughout my years studying orthopaedic implants, I discovered a significant divide between "the scientific aspects of joint replacements, academic research, and implant manufacturing", and "the availability of information accessible to patients and their families or caregivers".

However, initially I wasn't certain about the ways in which I could contribute to bridging this gap.

In late 2019, my beloved grandmother, Effat, underwent total knee replacement (TKA) surgery, and in early 2020, my dear mother-in-law, Karen, also had a TKA. This experience allowed me to witness first-hand the impact of joint replacement surgery on your loved ones and how it could affect the emotional well-being of you and your family, especially considering potential complications that might arise post-surgery.

That was when I made the decision to write this book. My goal was to share the knowledge I had accumulated over the years with everyone, with the hope of assisting those dealing with arthritis and those considering joint replacement as a solution for their hip or knee joint pain. My desire is for my readers to acquire a clearer comprehension of what a joint replacement entails and how it can impact a person's life.

I wrote this book with a diverse readership in mind. It's intended for a wide range of individuals, from those who are currently experiencing hip or knee pain, to individuals exploring the possibility of total hip or knee replacement for their ailment, as well as the families of patients. I would recommend this book for those who have undergone joint replacement surgery[1], those awaiting such a procedure, and the families and caregivers supporting them. Ultimately, I believe that anyone with an interest in orthopaedic implants will find value in reading this book.

Shahrzad, July 2020

The most recent edition includes some minor tweaks & additional information to facilitate better understanding of some of the technical concepts & topics covered in this book. Enjoy!

Shahrzad, October 2023

---

[1] The term 'joint replacement' in this book refers to both hip and knee replacement and is used when the information applies to both hips and knees.

Introduction

Within the pages of this book, you will find a concise exploration of the historical development of hip and knee replacements, with a particular focus on contemporary implant designs. We'll delve into the significance of considering hip and knee replacement options, explaining why the number of joint replacement surgeries has been steadily rising year after year.

In the second and third chapters of this book, we explore the specifics of hip and knee replacement implants, covering both current designs and the materials used for each component. Additionally, you'll find valuable information about the anatomy and biomechanics of the hip and knee joints.

Moving on to chapter four, you'll embark on an imaginary journey that starts a couple of days before your scheduled operation and concludes a few days after your discharge from the hospital. This segment is designed to provide insights into the preparations and arrangements required before surgery, offering a glimpse into the activities leading up to the day of the operation and the "behind-the-scenes" aspects of the process.

Towards the conclusion of this book, you'll discover five appendices, each serving a distinct purpose. These appendices encompass a "glossary" containing technical terms, phrases, and abbreviations from chapters one to four, "introducing gold-coloured hip and knee components", details on "body mass index (BMI)", and a handy "pre-surgery preparation checklist". It is my hope that these resources will prove valuable to you in your joint replacement journey.

Disclaimer 1 - The author of this book is not a licensed medical practitioner, and this book is intended solely for informational purposes and as a preliminary reference. It is strongly advised that readers consult a qualified orthopaedic consultant for personalised guidance. The author of this book disclaims any responsibility or liability for decisions made regarding joint replacement procedures solely based on the information contained in this book and without additional research. Readers are cautioned against taking any action based solely on the recommendations presented in this book & are encouraged to seek guidance from their healthcare provider, surgeon, or general physician, before making any decisions pertaining to their health, nutrition, or lifestyle.

Disclaimer 2 - The illustrations used in the book were obtained from the Microsoft Word Online Pictures pool. Most of these illustrations have an unknown author. In other words, the identity of the person or entity who created these illustrations is not known and (unless otherwise specified in the caption of any individual image or graph) the illustrations are licensed under CC BY (Creative Commons Attribution). This means that while the creator's identity is unknown, they have granted permission for others to use these illustrations in their own works, provided that proper attribution is given. CC BY allows for the free distribution, adaptation, and use of the illustrations as long as the original creator is credited.

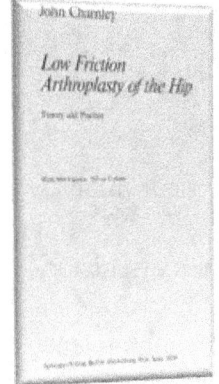
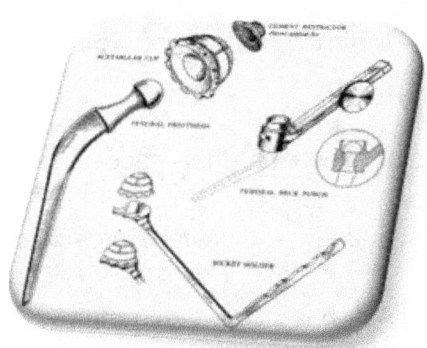

Chapter 1
A Historical Survey of Joint Replacement

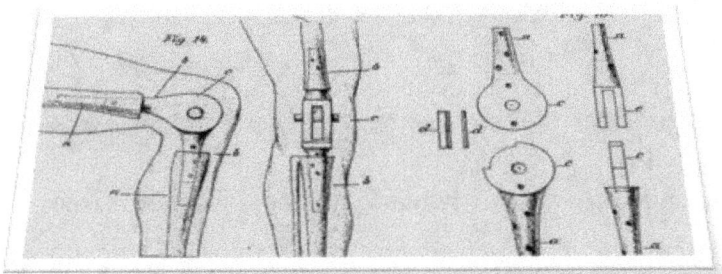

Chapter 1 - A Historical Survey of Joint Replacement

A Concise History of Joint Diseases

Joint diseases that cause pain and limit mobility have been a constant presence in human history, dating back to the emergence of anatomically modern humans approximately 200,000 years ago.

These conditions include arthritis, injuries, and various other musculoskeletal disorders that can affect the function of the joints.

In ancient times, when early humans were engaged in a hunter-gatherer lifestyle, the consequences of joint diseases were particularly significant.

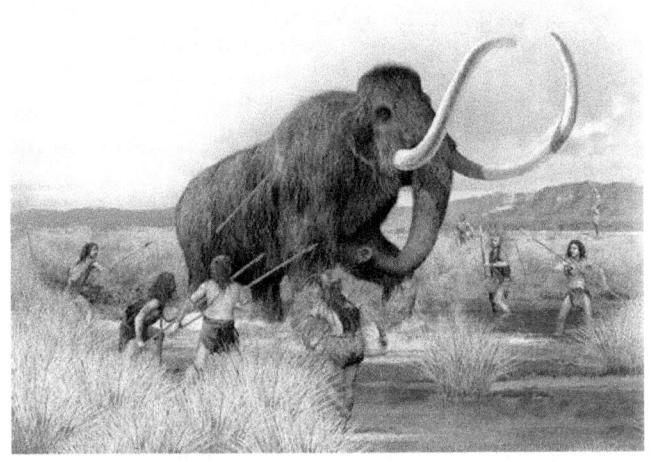

Figure 1-1 *Hunting woolly mammoth*

Early humans lived in a harsh and physically demanding environment. They relied on physical strength and mobility for activities like hunting, gathering, and carrying heavy prey or resources over long distances.

Joint diseases could made these activities extremely challenging, affecting an individual's ability to contribute to their community's survival.

Chapter 1 - A Historical Survey of Joint Replacement

In a hunter-gatherer society, the ability to move, walk, run, and carry loads was crucial for each individual's survival.

A painful and immobile joint, such as a knee, would have severely compromised a person's ability to hunt, forage for food, and escape from predators. In such situations, joint diseases could have life-threatening implications.

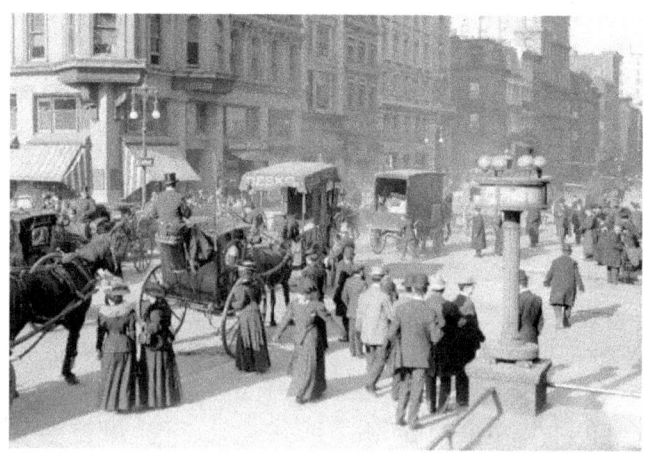

Figure 1-2 *Life in the 19th century*

Another significant contrast lies in life expectancy, which was notably lower in prehistoric and ancient societies, as well as during the Middle Ages, compared to the present day.

Back then many individuals did not live beyond their 30s or 40s due to a combination of factors, including infectious diseases, limited medical knowledge, and harsh living conditions.

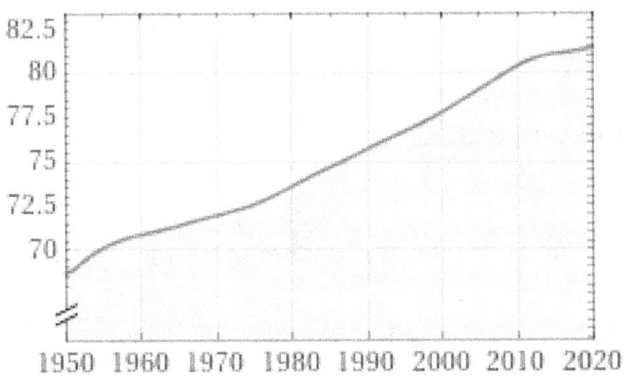

Figure 1-3 *Life expectancy history from 1950 to 2020 (United Kingdom) ©2023 WolframAlpha*

Chapter 1 - A Historical Survey of Joint Replacement

As a result, joint diseases may not have had the same long-term impact as they do in contemporary societies with longer life expectancies.

Historical Evidence of Joint Disease in Britain

One comprehensive research conducted in 1983 by Dr AK Thould's team at the Cornwall Department for Rheumatism Research, shed light on the prevalence of rheumatoid arthritis (RA) in ancient Roman Britain.

This study aimed to understand the patterns of arthritis in the Roman population living in Britain between 43 and 410 AD. To do so, the study examined the skeletal remains of 416 adult individuals from the Roman cemetery at Poundbury Camp, near Dorchester, Dorset.

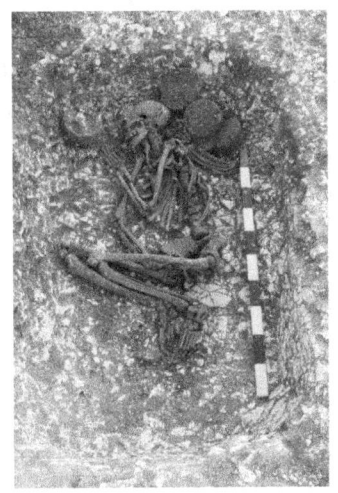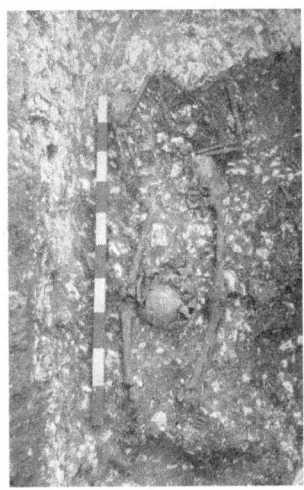

Figure 1-4 *Left: early Romano-British adult female, right: remains of a Romano-British decapitation burial of a juvenile, accompanied by a lamb ©2013 WessexArch*

The research findings revealed that rheumatoid arthritis was a notable health issue among the ancient Roman Britons.

Chapter 1 - A Historical Survey of Joint Replacement

Rheumatoid arthritis (RA) is a chronic autoimmune condition in which a person's immune system mistakenly attacks their own joints, leading to inflammation, pain, swelling, and stiffness. It can have a significant impact on an individual's quality of life and mobility. The presence of rheumatoid arthritis among the population of Roman Britain is historically significant for several reasons.

The study highlights that even in ancient times, people experienced and suffered from conditions like rheumatoid arthritis, demonstrating that such diseases have deep historical roots. This knowledge suggests that humans have been dealing with these health challenges for centuries.

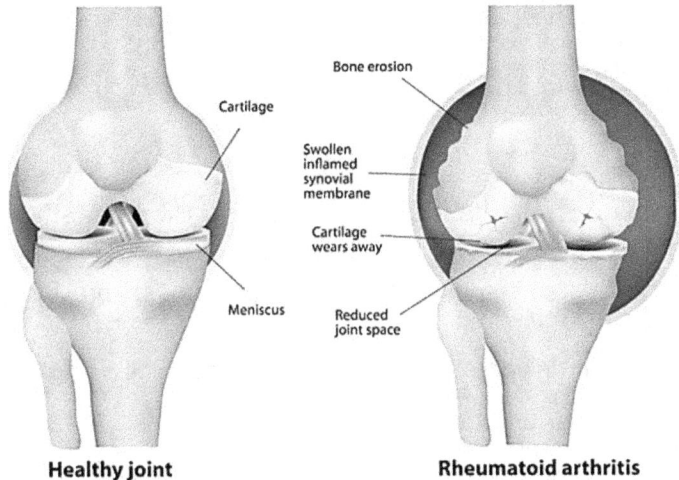

Figure 1-5 *Left: a healthy knee joint. Right: a knee joint affected by rheumatoid arthritis*

The findings also underscore the fact that individuals in ancient societies, including Roman Britain, faced significant health challenges that could affect their daily lives.

Rheumatoid arthritis, with its debilitating symptoms, would impact the ability to work, engage in daily activities, and participate in the community.

Research into ancient populations, like the study of skeletal remains from Roman times, provides valuable insights into the health and well-being of our ancestors.

It allows us to trace the prevalence of diseases, their impact on individuals, and the ways in which societies of the past may have coped with such health issues.

Historical Development of Surgical Principles

During the 18th and 19th centuries, significant advancements in surgical principles and techniques marked a pivotal moment in the history of orthopaedics and musculoskeletal medicine.

This era saw the establishment of surgical practices that revolutionised the treatment of bone fractures and joint conditions.

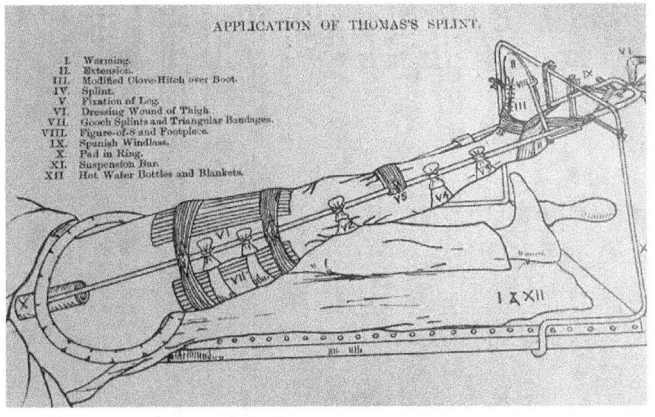

Figure 1-6 *Application of Thomas Splint - a common orthopaedic equipment in hospitals worldwide. First description by Hugh Owen Thomas published in 1875*

Setting and Fixing Fractures

Surgeons during this time began to develop standardised techniques for setting and immobilising fractured bones. The use of splints and casts became more refined, helping patients achieve better outcomes in fracture healing.

Alignment and Stability

Understanding the importance of aligning fractured bone ends correctly and ensuring stability played a crucial role in reducing complications and promoting proper bone healing.

However, these early endeavours faced significant challenges, primarily related to infection.

Infection was a major concern during this period because the principles of aseptic surgery (preventing infection through sterile techniques) were not yet fully understood or implemented.

The discovery of antibiotics, particularly penicillin, marked a transformative moment in the history of medicine and played a crucial role in addressing the significant challenges related to infection in early joint replacement surgeries.

Penicillin, one of the first widely used antibiotics, was discovered by Sir Alexander Fleming in 1928.

Chapter 1 - A Historical Survey of Joint Replacement

Fleming observed that the mould Penicillium chrysogenum produced a substance that could kill a wide range of bacteria.

This serendipitous discovery laid the foundation for the development of antibiotics, which proved to be a game-changer in the field of medicine.

Penicillin was first used in the 1940s, & its effectiveness in treating bacterial infections was nothing short of revolutionary.

The discovery and availability of antibiotics, especially penicillin, had a profound impact on joint arthroplasty. Surgeons could now administer antibiotics to patients before and after surgery, significantly reducing the risk of post-operative infections.

Prior to this development, joint replacement patients were vulnerable to various types of bacterial infections that could lead to serious complications, including implant failure.

With antibiotics, the risk of infection was substantially mitigated, allowing joint replacement surgery to become a safer and more effective procedure.

The discovery and widespread use of antibiotics also had broader implications for the entire field of medicine.

It revolutionised the treatment of various bacterial infections, making surgery safer, and improving patient outcomes in a wide range of medical procedures.

Antibiotics became an indispensable tool in modern medicine, and their impact on reducing infection rates in joint arthroplasty and other surgeries cannot be overstated.

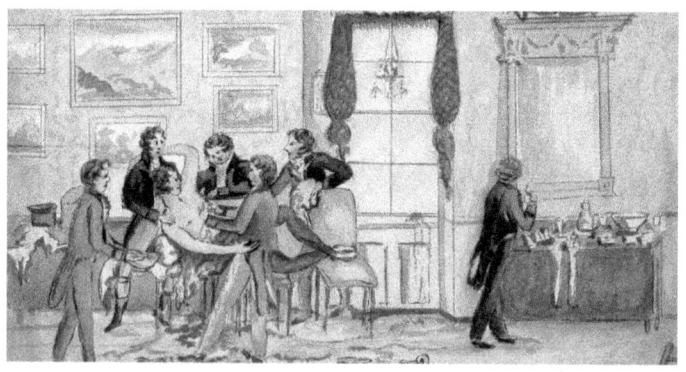

Figure 1-7 *An 18th century operating room*

Orthopaedic Surgery Advancements

Total Hip Replacement (THR)

THR is a surgical procedure that restores mobility and alleviates pain in individuals suffering from hip joint issues, represents a remarkable evolution in the field of orthopaedic medicine.

The history of THR is a testament to decades of innovation, surgical excellence, and a relentless commitment to improving the quality of life for patients.

Early Pioneering Efforts (19th to Early 20th Century) - The roots of total hip replacement can

Chapter 1 - A Historical Survey of Joint Replacement

be traced back to the late 19th century when pioneering surgeons began to experiment with hip joint surgeries.

However, it wasn't until the early 20th century that the concept of total hip replacement began to take shape.

One of the earliest recorded attempts was by Themistocles Gluck, who, in 1891, proposed the idea of using ivory to replace a hip joint, foreshadowing future developments in this field.

Innovations and Early Implants (1930s – 1950s) - The mid-20th century marked significant advancements in orthopaedic surgery, spurring the development of early hip implants.

Sir John Charnley, in the 1950s, introduced a groundbreaking design that included a cemented hip prosthesis. This innovation revolutionised hip replacement surgery and laid the foundation for modern THR.

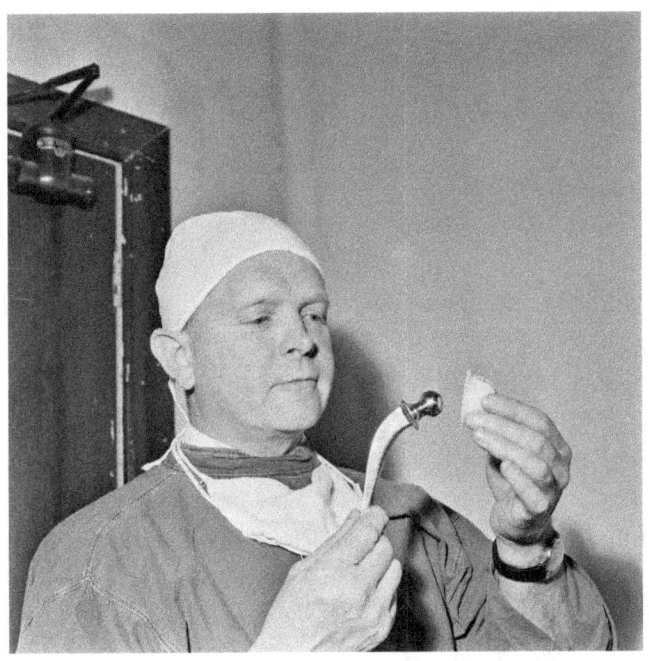

Figure 1-8 *Sir John Charnley at Wrightington Hospital (by Evening Standard/Getty Images)*

Chapter 1 - A Historical Survey of Joint Replacement

Advancements in Materials and Techniques (1960s – 1980s) - The 1960s to 1980s witnessed significant improvements in hip implant materials & surgical techniques.

Surgeons began experimenting with various materials like metal, ceramics, and newer forms of cement, aiming to enhance implant durability and reduce wear.

Minimally Invasive Approaches and Modern THR (1990s – Present) - The late 20th century saw the emergence of minimally invasive surgical techniques, which aimed to reduce patient trauma, blood loss, and recovery time.

These approaches, combined with advances in implant design and material science, have led to the development of modern THR procedures, providing patients with better outcomes and faster rehabilitation.

As THR continues to evolve, ongoing research explores innovative materials, improved implant designs, and the integration of advanced technologies like robotics.

The focus extends beyond surgical techniques to comprehensive post-operative care and patient education, ensuring individuals not only regain physical function but also achieve the best possible quality of life.

Total Knee Replacement (TKR)

TKR also known as total knee arthroplasty (TKA), is a groundbreaking achievement in modern medicine, transforming the lives of countless people with knee problems. Its history spans decades of innovation and dedication to improving patient well-being.

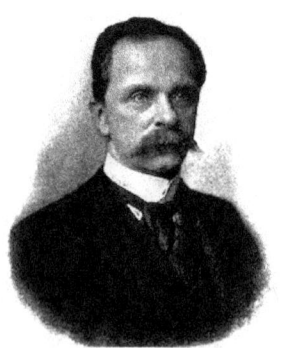

Figure 1-9 *Professor Themistocles Gluck (by Prof. Munjed Al Muderis)*

Early Beginnings (19th to Early 20th Century) - Total knee replacement traces its roots to the late 19th century when surgeons began experimenting with joint replacements.

In 1891, Themistocles Gluck suggested using ivory to replace a knee joint, laying the foundation for future developments.

Hinged Implants and Early Progress (1950s – 1970s) - In the mid-20th century, hinged knee implants gained traction.

Dr. Leslie Gordon Percival Shiers successfully implanted one in the 1950s, marking a shift away from total knee fusion. In the 1970s, Dr. John Insall and his colleagues developed the Insall-

Burstein knee prosthesis, setting the stage for modern knee replacement.

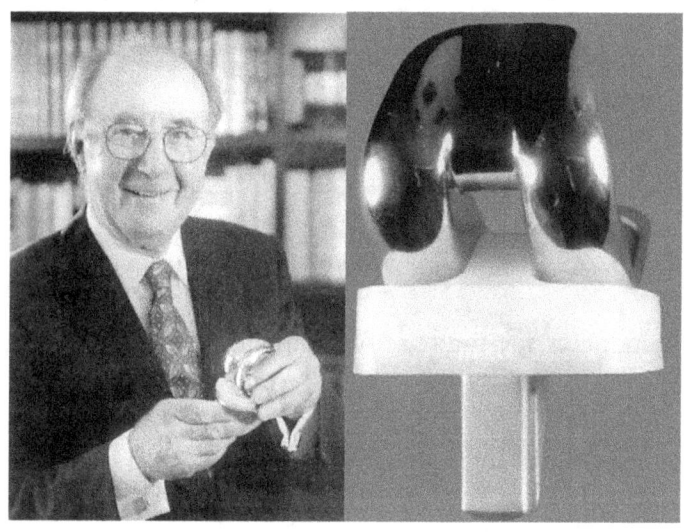

Figure 1-10 *Left: John Insall, MD. Right: the Insall Burstein Posterior Stabilised I Knee prosthesis was designed to substitute for the posterior cruciate ligament (Giles R. Scuderi, MD)*

Implant Advancements and Surgical Techniques (1980s – 1990s) - The 1980s and 1990s brought material improvements and minimally invasive surgery techniques, enhancing implant durability and patient recovery.

Computer Assistance and Personalised Implants (2000s – Present) - The 2000s introduced computer-assisted surgeries and personalised implants, increasing precision and tailoring solutions to patients' anatomy.

Current Trends and Future Prospects - Research now explores innovative materials and robotic-assisted surgeries for even greater precision.

Multidisciplinary approaches encompassing rehabilitation and patient well-being.

Groundbreaking Advancements in Joint Surgery

Anthony White, an orthopaedic surgeon at Westminster Hospital in London, is notable for his pioneering work in joint arthroplasty. In 1822, he performed a groundbreaking procedure known as "excision joint arthroplasty".

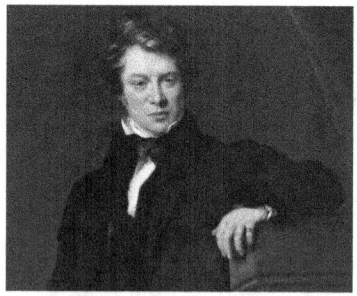

Figure 1-11 *Professor Anthony White (by Chelsea and Westminster Hospital)*

This technique involved removing the diseased parts of a joint, allowing the body to naturally replace the excised tissue with scar tissue.

Anthony White's approach represented a significant departure from early attempts at implanting artificial joints.

Instead of inserting prosthetic materials, he relied on the body's natural healing process to form scar tissue, providing stability and pain relief to the affected joint.

Anthony White's excision joint arthroplasty was a pivotal development in the history of joint surgery for several reasons some of which are listed below.

Chapter 1 - A Historical Survey of Joint Replacement

Infection Control:

By not introducing foreign materials into the joint, the risk of infection was significantly reduced, addressing one of the main challenges faced by early attempts at artificial joints.

Preservation of Function:

While scar tissue may not fully replicate the function of the original joint, it often provided a level of stability and pain relief that improved the patient's quality of life.

Foundation for Future Advances:

White's work laid the foundation for future advancements in joint surgery, eventually leading to the development of modern joint replacement techniques.

The late 18th century and the subsequent decades witnessed significant innovations in implant materials and surgical techniques.

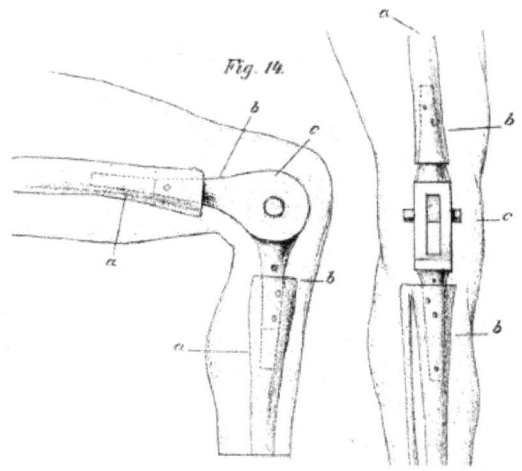

Figure 1-12 *Biographical sketch: Themistocles Gluck (1853–1942)* © *SpringerLink*

These developments laid the groundwork for modern joint replacement surgery. During this time, surgeons and inventors were exploring various materials and designs for artificial joints.

Chapter 1 - A Historical Survey of Joint Replacement

Professor Themistocles Gluck (1853 – 1942), a renowned orthopaedic surgeon from Berlin, played a pivotal role in the early history of joint arthroplasty. Professor Gluck is credited with introducing the term "arthroplasty" in 1902.

Arthroplasty refers to the surgical reconstruction or replacement of a joint. In 1890, Professor Gluck performed one of the earliest recorded cases of implanting an artificial knee joint.

This marked a significant advancement in the field of joint surgery. Professor Gluck's pioneering work extended to hip joint surgery. In 1891, he implanted the world's first artificial hip joint. His design utilised an ivory head fixed to the bone with a nickel plate and screws, representing an early attempt at hip arthroplasty.

Acrylic implants were another significant development in the history of joint replacement. Notably, the Judet brothers from Paris, Robert and Jean Judet, contributed to the success of acrylic implants.

In 1948, Robert and Jean Judet introduced acrylic implants for the replacement of the femoral head in hip joints. These implants gained popularity due to their durability and biocompatibility.

The Judet brothers' acrylic implant is known for its exceptional in vivo durability. It holds the world record for lasting 51 years inside a patient's body, demonstrating its long-term success and effectiveness.

The contributions of Professor Gluck and the Judet brothers marked critical milestones in the evolution of joint arthroplasty.

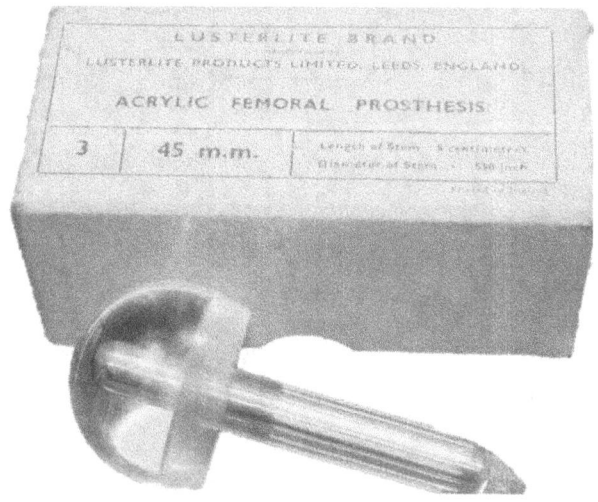

Figure 1-13 *Judet acrylic femoral head (by Dr Prakash)*

Their work not only expanded the possibilities of joint replacement but also paved the way for the development of more advanced and long-lasting implant materials and surgical techniques in the decades that followed.

During the same timeframe, advancements in artificial knee development were underway, but their success rates lagged behind those of hip implants.

The relatively lower success rate of artificial knees was not solely attributed to the choice of implant design and materials. The low success rate of artificial knees was also significantly influenced by challenges related to surgical techniques and inadequate joint stability.

Chapter 1 - A Historical Survey of Joint Replacement

Unlike the hip joint, which benefited from more straightforward anatomy and biomechanics, the knee joint presented a considerably more intricate structural and functional complexity.

The knee joint's complexity arises from its unique anatomy and the intricate network of soft tissues that surround and support it.

The intricate nature of this complexity presented unique challenges for orthopaedic surgeons, which will be explored in chapter three.

The complexity also posed distinct challenges for implant designers, leading to a more complex and nuanced set of issues that needed to be addressed for successful knee surgery outcomes.

Total Joint Replacement or Arthroplasty

Joint replacement, also known as joint arthroplasty, is a surgical procedure that involves the replacement of a damaged, painful, or dysfunctional joint with an artificial prosthesis.

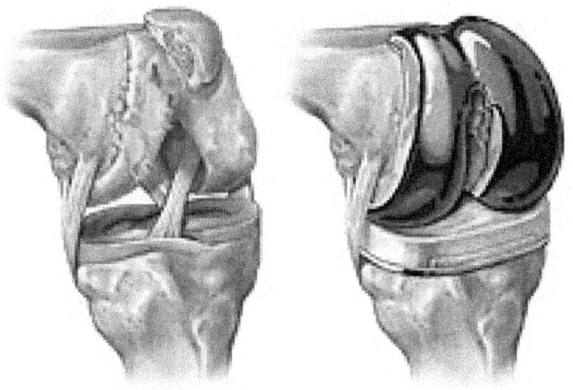

Figure 1-14 *Left: an unhealthy & painful knee joint, right: a total knee joint replacement (by ADAM)*

Chapter 1 - A Historical Survey of Joint Replacement

This procedure is commonly performed on major weight-bearing joints like the hip and knee, as well as the shoulder.

It can also be applied to other joints such as the ankle, elbow, and wrist, depending on the patient's condition and need.

Joint replacement is a medical intervention primarily used to relieve pain, improve joint function, and enhance the patient's overall quality of life.

It is typically recommended for individuals who have severe joint conditions, often due to osteoarthritis, rheumatoid arthritis, traumatic injuries, or congenital disorders.

In joint replacement surgery, the damaged or diseased parts of the joint are removed, and they are replaced with especially designed prosthetic components.

These prosthetic components are engineered to mimic the natural movement and function of the joint as closely as possible.

Joint replacement surgery aims to alleviate pain, restore joint mobility, and allow patients to return to their normal activities.

Performing normal activities including walking, climbing stairs, and performing daily tasks, without the limitations imposed by a painful or damaged joint.

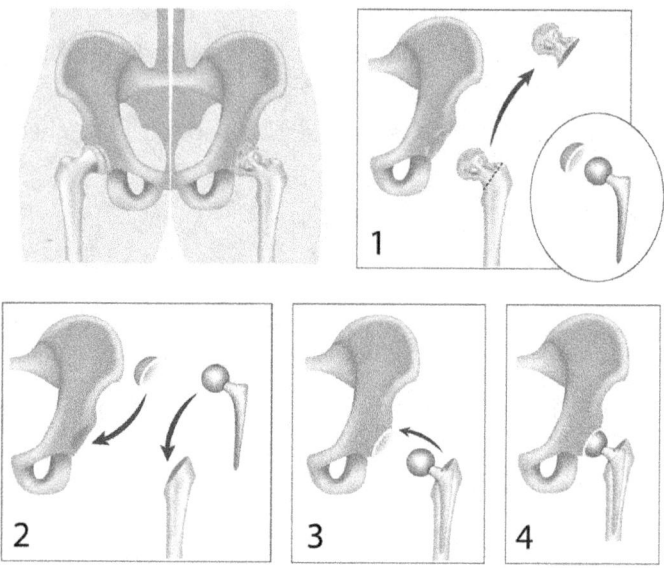

Figure 1-15 *Hip prosthetic components engineered to mimic the natural movement and function of the joint as closely as possible (by Alila Medical Images / Alamy Stock Photo)*

Prior to undergoing joint replacement surgery, patients undergo a thorough evaluation by medical professionals.

This assessment includes reviewing the patient's medical history, conducting imaging tests, and assessing the overall health and fitness of the patient to determine their suitability for the surgery.

Following joint replacement surgery, patients typically engage in a structured rehabilitation program.

This includes physical therapy exercises to strengthen the joint, improve range of motion, and aid in a speedy recovery.

Rehabilitation plays a critical role in achieving the best possible outcomes.

Chapter 1 - A Historical Survey of Joint Replacement

The concept of joints losing function due to wear and tear, much like other aspects of the body deteriorating with age, is a fundamental aspect of musculoskeletal health.

Joints are the critical points in our body where bones meet and allow movement.

Over the course of a lifetime, these joints are subjected to continuous use and mechanical stress. This daily wear and tear gradually affect their structure and function.

The degree of wear and tear can vary from person to person and can be influenced by various factors, including genetics, lifestyle, and environmental factors.

The most common condition associated with the wear and tear of joints is osteoarthritis (OA).

OA is a degenerative joint disease that primarily affects older individuals, although it can also develop in younger people with certain risk factors.

In OA, the cartilage that cushions the ends of bones in a joint gradually deteriorates or breaks down.

This loss of cartilage leads to pain, swelling, stiffness, and a reduction in joint function. Over time, OA can cause significant joint damage and impact a person's ability to perform daily activities.

Chapter 1 - A Historical Survey of Joint Replacement

Rheumatoid arthritis (RA) is a chronic autoimmune condition that significantly differs from the wear and tear of joints seen in osteoarthritis (OA).

While OA primarily affects older individuals, RA can strike at any age.

In RA, the body's immune system mistakenly attacks the synovium, the lining of the membranes that surround the joints.

This relentless assault causes inflammation, which, over time, erodes the cartilage and damages the joint.

The result is pain, swelling, stiffness, and often deformities in the affected joints.

Osteoarthritis and rheumatoid arthritis

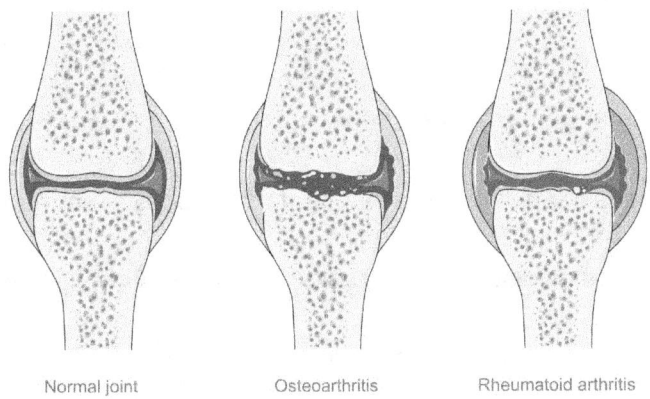

Normal joint   Osteoarthritis   Rheumatoid arthritis

Figure 1-16 *A normal, OA, and RA joint*

RA can have a profound impact on a person's quality of life, affecting their mobility and daily activities.

Early diagnosis and appropriate treatment are crucial in managing RA and minimising joint damage. Other differences between RA and OA are listed next.

- Rheumatoid arthritis (RA) vs osteoarthritis (OA) causes:

Rheumatoid Arthritis or RA is an autoimmune disease, which means that the body's immune system mistakenly attacks healthy joint tissues, primarily the synovium (the lining of the membranes that surround the joints). The exact cause of RA is not known, but it is believed to result from a combination of genetic, environmental, and hormonal factors.

Osteoarthritis (OA) is primarily a degenerative joint disease. It occurs when the protective cartilage that cushions the ends of bones breaks down over time. OA is often associated with ageing, joint overuse, and joint injuries.

- Rheumatoid arthritis (RA) vs osteoarthritis (OA) location of joint involvement:

RA typically affects multiple joints symmetrically, meaning it simultaneously impacts corresponding joints on both sides of the body. Commonly affected joints include the wrists, knees, fingers, and toes. This symmetrical pattern is a distinguishing feature of RA.

Osteoarthritis (OA) primarily affects weight-bearing joints like the knees, hips, spine, and hands due to the mechanical wear and tear these joints endure over time. Managing OA involves pain relief, lifestyle adjustments, physical therapy, and, in some cases, surgical interventions.

- Rheumatoid arthritis (RA) vs osteoarthritis (OA) symptoms:

RA symptoms include joint pain, swelling, and stiffness, which are usually worse in the morning or after periods of inactivity. Fatigue, fever, and general malaise. RA can also lead to joint deformities over time.

In OA symptoms are joint pain that worsens with activity and improves with rest. Stiffness after periods of inactivity but typically improves with movement. Joint crepitus (a cracking or grating sensation) may occur.

- Rheumatoid arthritis (RA) vs osteoarthritis (OA) diagnosis:

RA diagnosis often involves blood tests to check for specific antibodies like rheumatoid factor (RF) and anti-citrullinated protein antibodies (ACPAs).

OA diagnosis is usually based on physical examination and imaging tests like X-rays. Blood tests are not typically used for diagnosing OA.

- Rheumatoid arthritis (RA) vs osteoarthritis (OA) treatment methods and options:

Rheumatoid arthritis treatment usually focuses on suppressing the autoimmune response with medications like disease-modifying anti-rheumatic drugs (DMARDs) and biologics. Pain relief is often provided with non-steroidal anti-inflammatory drugs (NSAIDs) and corticosteroids.

Whereas OA treatment aims to manage pain and improve joint function. This can include lifestyle modifications, physical therapy, pain medications (such as NSAIDs), and sometimes joint injections. In severe cases, joint replacement surgery may be recommended.

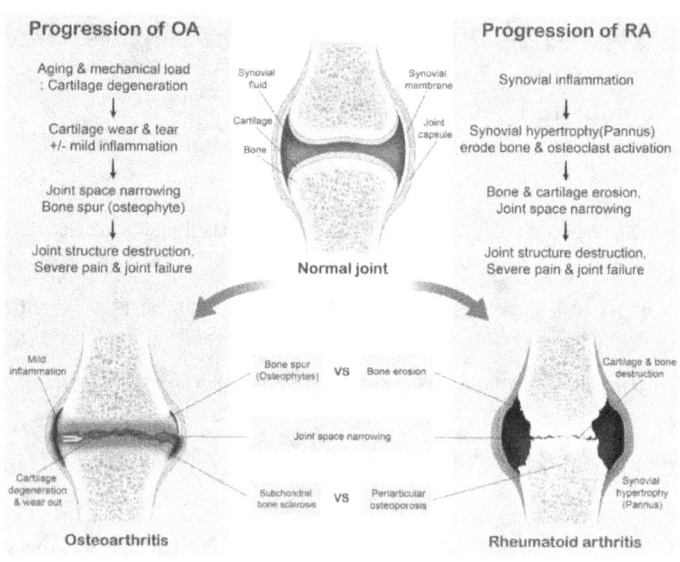

Figure 1-17 *OA vs RA*

In general, several factors contribute to the wear and tear of joints, some of the most important contributing factors are listed below.

Age:

The natural ageing process plays a significant role. As we age, the body's ability to repair and maintain joint tissues diminishes, making joints more susceptible to degeneration.

BMI:

Excess body weight places increased stress on weight-bearing joints, such as the knees and hips, accelerating the degenerative process.

Injury:

Chapter 1 - A Historical Survey of Joint Replacement

Previous joint injuries or trauma can contribute to the development of OA in specific joints.

Repetition:

Joints that are frequently used or subjected to repetitive motions are more prone to wear and tear. This is common in occupations or activities that involve heavy lifting, repetitive bending, or high-impact activities.

Genetics:

Some people may have a genetic predisposition to joint problems, making them more susceptible to degeneration. While joint wear and tear are natural parts of the ageing process, there are ways to manage and mitigate its impact.

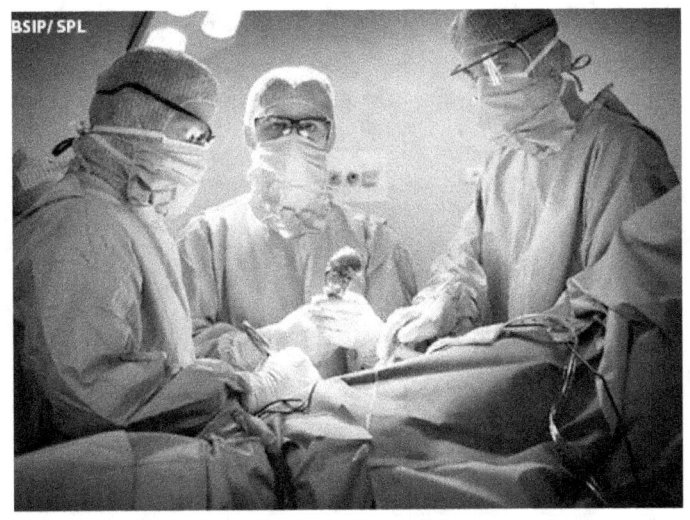

Figure 1-18 *Joint replacement surgery*

For example by maintaining a healthy weight, staying physically active, and avoiding excessive repetitive movements you can help reduce the risk of joint deterioration.

Also anti-inflammatory medications and pain relievers may be prescribed to manage joint pain and inflammation.

Chapter 1 - A Historical Survey of Joint Replacement

Remember, physical therapy exercises can help strengthen the muscles around the affected joint, improve joint stability, and alleviate symptoms; and of course, in cases of severe joint degeneration or severe joint pain that significantly impairs quality of life, joint replacement surgery, as discussed earlier, can provide effective relief.

Joint Replacements in Contemporary Times

Let's delve into the topic of global life expectancy and compare statistical data from the current time to approximately 70 years ago when modern designs of hip and knee replacements were taking shape.

Global life expectancy is a measure of how long, on average, people in a given population can expect to live.

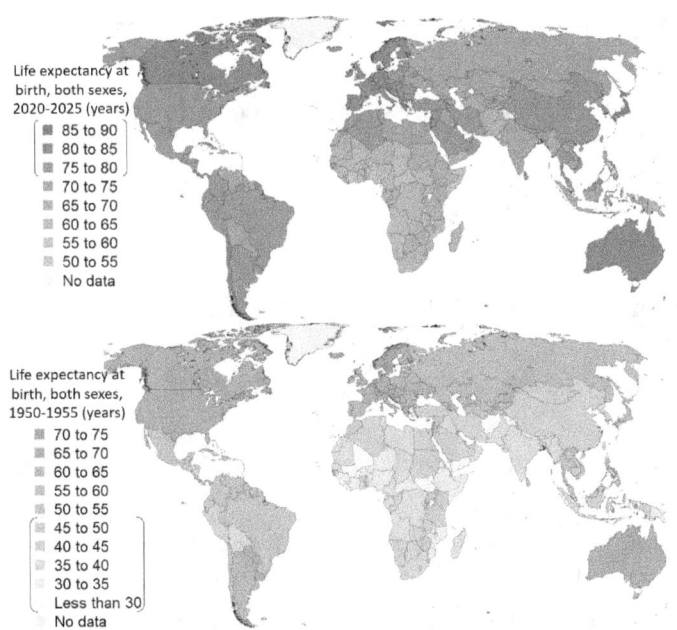

Figure 1-19 *Top: life expectancy in 2020-2025, bottom: life expectancy in 1950-1955 ©2019 UN*

It is a critical indicator of a nation's overall health and reflects improvements in healthcare, living standards, nutrition, sanitation, and medical advancements. Life expectancy varies by country and has seen substantial changes over the years.

Around 70 years ago, in the 1950s, life expectancy worldwide was considerably lower than it is today.

Several factors contributed to this. In the 1950s, many countries were still grappling with high mortality rates from infectious diseases such as tuberculosis, influenza, and pneumonia. These diseases posed significant threats to public health.

Furthermore, there was high child mortality rates, primarily due to infectious diseases and lack of access to proper healthcare and nutrition, which influenced overall life expectancy.

In addition, medical advancements, including those related to joint replacement surgery, were in their infancy. Hip and knee replacements as we know them today are still in the experimental stages and not widely available.

Fast-forward to the 2020s, and we see a vastly different global landscape in terms of life expectancy.

Advances in vaccination, antibiotics, & healthcare infrastructure have led to a substantial reduction in mortality from infectious diseases. Many

Chapter 1 - A Historical Survey of Joint Replacement

countries have successfully controlled or eliminated these once-devastating illnesses.

Child mortality rates have significantly decreased due to better access to healthcare, improved nutrition, and increased awareness of maternal & child health.

Medical technology and surgical techniques have advanced dramatically, including joint replacement surgery.

Modern joint replacements, with improved materials and surgical methods, have become highly successful procedures, providing relief to millions of people suffering from joint diseases.

Comparing life expectancy between the 1950s and the 2020s, we see a substantial increase in the average lifespan globally. While specific data may vary by region and country, the overall trend is one of improvement.

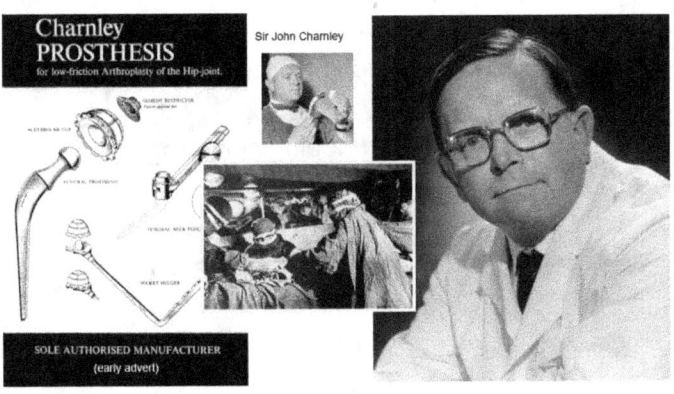

Figure 1-20 *First modern hip replacement (low friction prostheses) by Sir John Charnley*

In many developed countries today, life expectancy is well into the 70s, 80s, or even

90s. This increase in life expectancy has several implications:

- People are living longer, and as a result, there is a growing ageing population.

- Chronic diseases and degenerative joint conditions, which become more prevalent with age, are a significant health concern.

- The demand for medical interventions like joint replacement surgery has surged, as individuals seek ways to maintain mobility and quality of life in their later years.

According to the United Nations (UN), ageing is indeed a global issue. *"The world population is ageing, and virtually every country in the world is experiencing growth in the number and proportion of older persons in their population.*

Population ageing is poised to become one of the most significant social transformations of the twenty-first century.

There is increasing consideration of older persons as contributors to development. There is also an acknowledgement that this demographic contributes to the betterment of themselves and their societies.

Therefore, we need to weave their needs into policies and programmes at all levels. As a result, in the coming decades, many countries are likely to face fiscal and political pressures

Chapter 1 - A Historical Survey of Joint Replacement

about public systems of health care, pensions, and social protection for a growing older population".

In contemporary society, there has been a noticeable shift towards a more sedentary lifestyle for various reasons. Modern technology has brought about a range of conveniences, such as delivery services for food, groceries, and online shopping.

These services reduce the need for physical activity associated with going to the store or preparing meals. The proliferation of digital entertainment, including gaming consoles and other electronic devices, has led to a shift in recreational activities.

Many children & teenagers now spend more time indoors engaging in digital entertainment rather than outdoor physical activities like street football.

The reduction in physical activity associated with these lifestyle changes has several consequences, as with less need to move about for daily tasks, people are becoming less mobile. This can result in a decline in overall physical fitness and agility.

Reduced physical activity can contribute to various health issues, including (but not limited to) obesity, cardiovascular problems, and musculoskeletal conditions.

Also, prolonged periods of sitting can lead to posture-related pain & musculoskeletal problems.

Chapter 1 - A Historical Survey of Joint Replacement

The preference for indoor digital entertainment among children and teenagers can limit their opportunities for physical play and exercise. This can have long-term implications for their physical and mental health.

Another important factor to consider is nutrition. The availability and convenience of low-quality, fast food options have led to changes in dietary habits.

Fast food tends to be high in calories, saturated fats, and sugars while lacking essential nutrients. Consuming such foods regularly can contribute to weight gain and overall poor nutrition.

The combination of reduced physical activity and poor nutrition has led to an increase in the average weight of individuals in many parts of the world; & obesity rates have risen significantly.

As mentioned, the combination of reduced mobility, sedentary lifestyles, and poor nutrition can have wide-ranging health implications.

Obesity is a major public health concern, as it is associated with an increased risk of chronic conditions like diabetes, heart disease, and joint problems.

Reduced physical activity can also impact mental health, potentially contributing to issues like stress and depression.

Chapter 1 - A Historical Survey of Joint Replacement

The decline in mobility and overall physical fitness can affect an individual's quality of life, limiting their ability to engage in daily activities and enjoy a full range of experiences.

BMI is a widely used measurement that assesses an individual's body weight in relation to their height. It's a simple formula that helps gauge whether a person's weight falls within a "healthy range".

The BMI formula is calculated by dividing an individual's weight (in kilograms) by the square of their height (in meters). The resulting number is the BMI score.

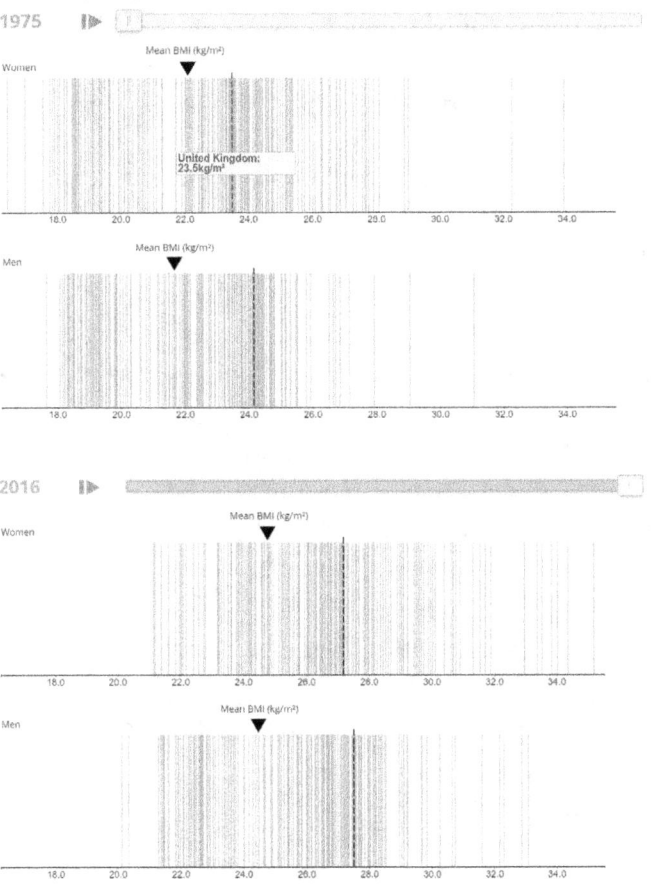

Figure 1-21 *The mean BMI, from top to bottom: women in 1975 (22), men in 1975 (21.5), women in 2016 (25) & men in 2016 (24.5). Note the dotted line indicates average BMI in the UK*
©2017 NCD Risk Factor Collaboration

To understand the global trends in weight gain and obesity over the years, comparing mean BMI scores for women and men worldwide can be quite informative.

The mean BMI score is an average of all individual BMI scores in a particular group, in this case, women and men globally.

The comparison of mean BMI scores for women and men between 1975 and 2016 highlights a significant trend.

In this context, a rising mean BMI score indicates that, on average, people in these groups have been gaining weight over the years.

The increase in mean BMI scores is indicative of a global trend toward higher body weights among both women and men.

Several factors have contributed to the rise in mean BMI scores over the decades, including changes in dietary habits, reduced physical activity, and increased consumption of calorie-dense foods.

An increase in mean BMI scores is often associated with a higher prevalence of overweight and obesity within a population.

High BMI levels are linked to a greater risk of various health problems, including cardiovascular diseases, type 2 diabetes, certain cancers, and musculoskeletal issues.

It also places additional strain on healthcare systems due to the increased demand for medical services related to obesity-related conditions.

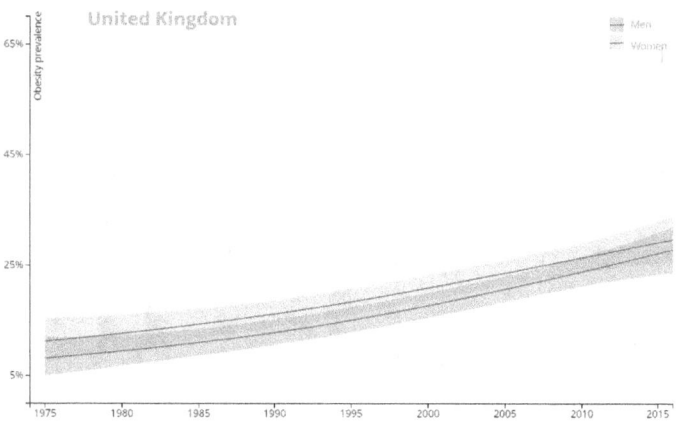

Figure 1-22 *Obesity prevalence in the UK between the years 1975 and 2016 separated by gender ©2017 NCD Risk Factor Collaboration*

One's BMI score typically falls within the range of 18.5 to 30, and an increase in weight is usually accompanied by an increase in the BMI score.

According to the United Nations (UN), an individual with a BMI score below 18.5 is classified as underweight, while a BMI score exceeding 30 indicates obesity.

Currently, there is a substantial and rapid increase in obesity within the UK population over the past four decades.

There is significant impact of one's weight on the progression of joint diseases, particularly in weight-bearing joints like the hips.

Chapter 1 - A Historical Survey of Joint Replacement

When an individual walks, the forces exerted on their joints, for example, on the hip joint, are directly influenced by their body weight.

Factors like increased weight, walking speed, or walking on an incline can further increase the pressure on the joints.

This underscores that lifestyle factors and conditions affecting body weight and activity level can have a direct impact on joint health.

To better understand the increasing prevalence of joint replacement procedures, I delved into the data from the 16th annual report of the UK National Joint Registry (NJR), which was published in 2020.

As confirmed by Professor Mike Reed, the Chairman of the NJR Editorial Board, this annual report draws from a vast pool of 2,835,101 records, solidifying NJR's position as the foremost global source of registry data.

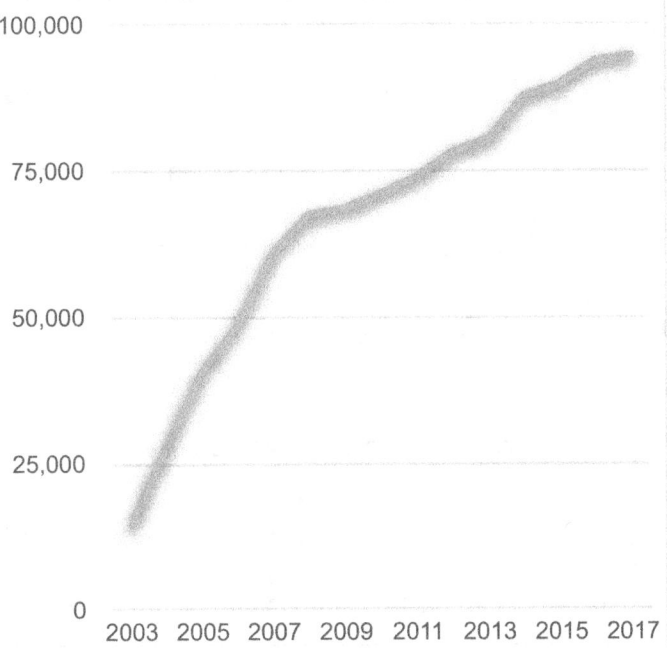

Figure 1-23 *An increase in the rate of primary total hip replacement operations*

Chapter 1 - A Historical Survey of Joint Replacement

One of the factors that plays a role in shaping the development of joint replacement procedures, even though it may not seem immediately apparent, is the influence of sports-related injuries. This also applies to professional dancers and performers.

In the broader context, a person's activity level serves as a significant risk factor in joint health. To gauge this activity level more precisely, there is a system available (example below).

Tegner Activity Scale provides a succinct assessment by evaluating an individual's engagement in both occupational and sports activities, assigning a rating on a scale from zero to ten.

10 Competitive sports-soccer, football, rugby (national elite)
9   Competitive sports-soccer, football, rugby (lower divisions), ice hockey, wrestling, gymnastics, basketball
8   Competitive sports-racquetball, squash or badminton, track and field athletics (jumping, etc.), downhill skiing
7   Competitive sports-tennis, running, motorcars speedway, handball
    Recreational sports-soccer, football, rugby, ice-hockey, basketball, squash, racquetball, running
6   Recreational sports-tennis and badminton, handball, racquetball, downhill skiing, jogging at least 5 x per week
5   Work-heavy labor (construction, etc.)
    Competitive sports-cycling, cross-country skiing
    Recreational sports-jogging on uneven ground at least twice weekly
4   Work-moderately heavy labor (e.g. truck driving, etc.)
    Recreational sports-cycling, cross-country skiing, jogging on even ground at least twice weekly
3   Work-light labor (nursing, etc.)
    Competitive and recreational sports-swimming, walking in forest possible
2   Walking on uneven ground possible, but impossible to back pack or hike
1   Work-sedentary (secretarial, etc.)
0   Sick leave or disability pension because of knee problems

Figure 1-24 *The activity scale for knee joint, levels 0 to 10*

A score of zero on this scale indicates a state of disability due to knee or hip issues, while a score of ten signifies active participation in competitive sports at either the national or international level.

Bilateral Joint Arthroplasty

Before moving on to the next chapter, let's have a quick look at what "bilateral joint replacement" is. Bilateral joint replacement, also known as bilateral arthroplasty, refers to the surgical procedure in which both joints in a pair (such as both hips or both knees) are replaced.

This can be during a single surgical session (simultaneous bilateral hip/knee replacement or in a staged bilateral replacement, both joints (hips or knees) are replaced in two separate surgeries which are usually done a few months apart. It can be bilateral total hip replacement (BTHR), bilateral total knee replacement (BTKR), or even involve other joints like the shoulders or ankles.

Bilateral joint replacement is typically recommended for patients who have severe joint degeneration, pain, and limited mobility in both joints simultaneously.

This approach is considered when both joints are affected to a significant extent, and it's more practical and efficient to address both at once rather than having two separate surgeries.

One of the primary advantages of bilateral joint replacement is that it allows for a single recovery period. Instead of going through the rehabilitation and recovery process twice for each joint, the patient can focus on healing from both surgeries simultaneously.

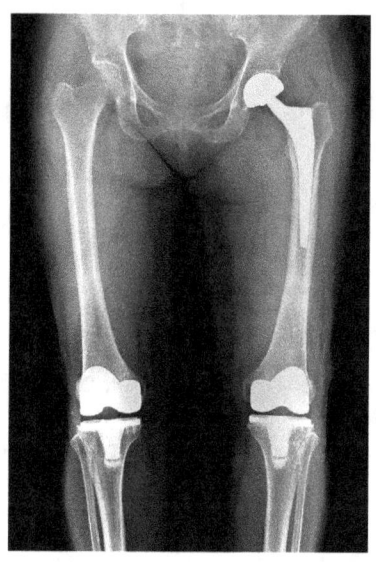

Figure 1-25 *Bilateral TKR and unilateral (left side) THR (by ChooChin / Getty Images)*

Also, since both joints are addressed in one surgical session, the patient undergoes anaesthesia only once, which can reduce the overall risks associated with anaesthesia.

In addition, the hospital stay may be shorter compared to having two separate surgeries. Bilateral joint replacement can be more cost-effective than having two separate procedures since it consolidates some of the costs associated with surgery, hospitalisation, and rehabilitation.

Bilateral joint replacement is a more complex procedure than unilateral (single) joint replacement. It requires more time in the operating room and demands a high level of surgical skill and precision.

Because of the increased surgical complexity, there may be a slightly higher risk of complications, such as blood clots, infections, and cardiac issues. However, these risks are often carefully managed by the surgical team.

While the recovery process is consolidated, it can be more challenging for the patient, as both joints are recovering simultaneously. Physical therapy and rehabilitation are crucial for regaining mobility and function.

Not all patients are candidates for bilateral joint replacement. Factors such as the patient's overall health, age, and the severity of joint disease play a role in determining whether this approach is appropriate.

A thorough evaluation by a healthcare team, including an orthopaedic surgeon, is essential to assess the patient's candidacy.

After bilateral joint replacement, patients typically follow a structured rehabilitation plan. This includes physical therapy to improve joint function and strength. Pain management is also a critical aspect of post-operative care.

As such, bilateral arthroplasty comes with increased surgical complexity and considerations regarding patient selection and post-operative care. It is a viable option for individuals who have significant joint issues in both joints and are deemed suitable candidates by their healthcare team.

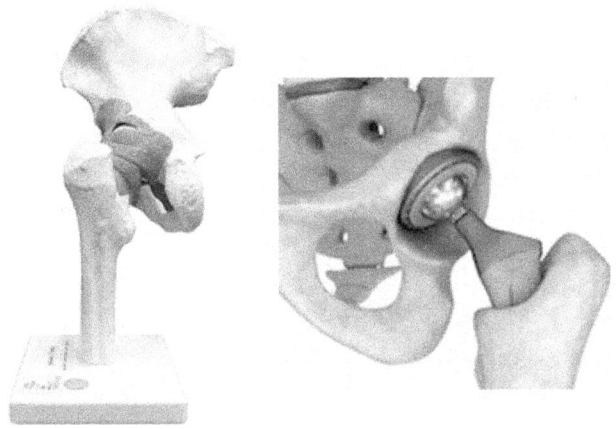

Chapter 2
The Hip Joint

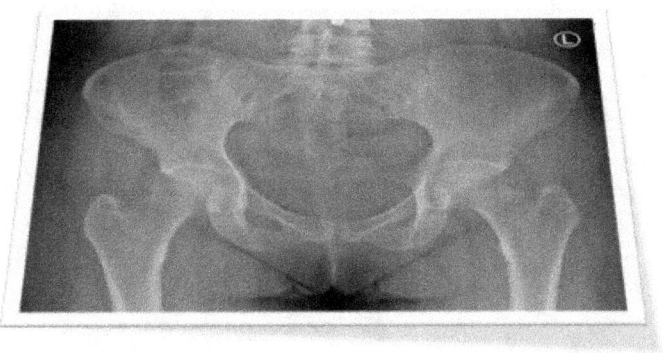

Chapter 2 - The Hip Joint

An Introduction to the Hip Joint

In this section, we will provide a concise overview of the essential characteristics and functions of the hip joint.

The hip joint is classified as a ball-and-socket joint, enabling movement through the interaction between the head of the femur (thigh bone) and the acetabulum socket located within the pelvis.

Before progressing to the subsequent section, let us familiarise ourselves with some common anatomical terms.

Anatomical Planes & Motion Axes

To enhance our comprehension of bone and joint structures and movements, it's beneficial to familiarise ourselves with three reference anatomical planes and three motion axes.

These references serve as valuable tools for clearer explanations.

- Transverse or Axial Plane (also known as the Horizontal Plane): This plane separates the body into superior and inferior (top and bottom) portions, providing a critical perspective on anatomical structures.

Chapter 2 - The Hip Joint

- Sagittal or Longitudinal Plane: This is an imaginary plane that divides the body or a bone into left and right parts.

- Coronal or Frontal Plane: This plane bisects the body into front and back sides, aiding in visualising movements and orientations.

In conjunction with these planes, there are three motion axes:

- Craniocaudal Axis: This axis represents movement from head to toe or vice versa.

- Anteroposterior Axis: Accounts for movements occurring from front to back or back to front.

- Left-Right Axis: This axis signifies movements in a lateral direction, left to right or right to left.

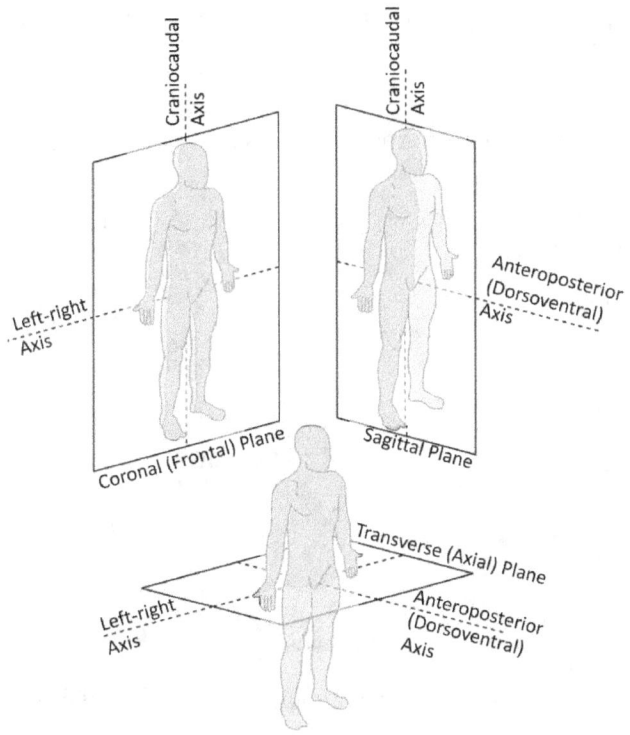

Figure 2-1 *Anatomical reference planes and axes*

These anatomical planes & motion axes serve as valuable reference points in understanding the complexities of bone/joint functions & movements.

Chapter 2 - The Hip Joint

Anatomy and Biomechanics of the Hip Joint

The hip joint boasts a remarkable range of motion, owing to its unique shape and physical attributes.

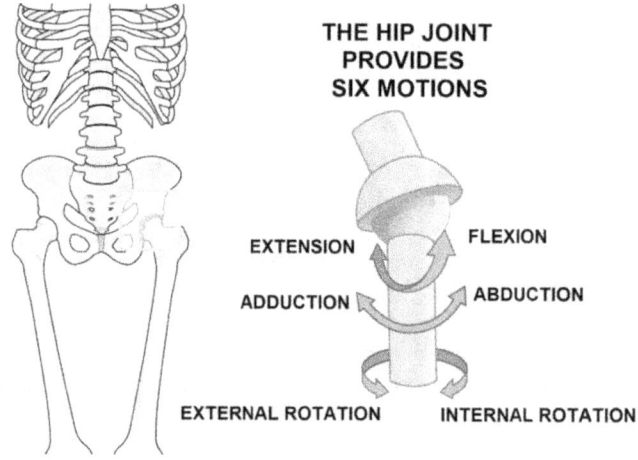

Figure 2-2 *The hip joint provides the following movements: abduction, adduction, flexion, extension and internal and external rotation*

Table 2-1 *Summary of the hip kinematics*

Motion	Normal range of motion degrees	Plane of motion
Flexion	0-120	
Extension	0-120	
Abduction	0-40	
Adduction	0-25	
Internal Rotation	0-35	
External Rotation	0-45	

Chapter 2 - The Hip Joint

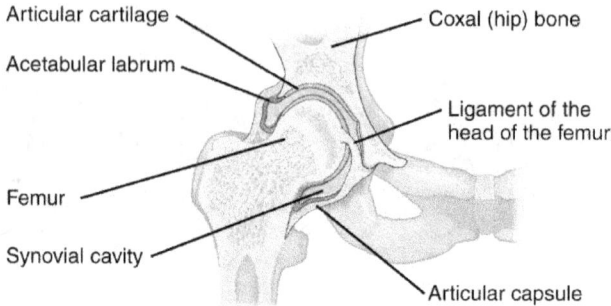

(a) Frontal section through the right hip joint

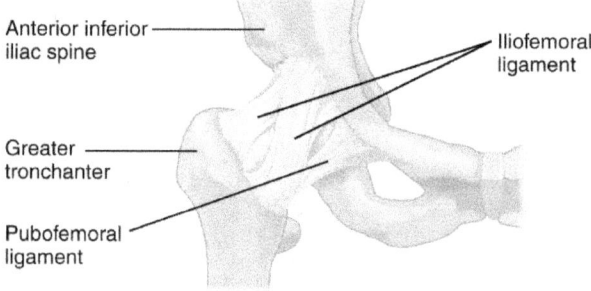

(b) Anterior view of right hip joint, capsule in place

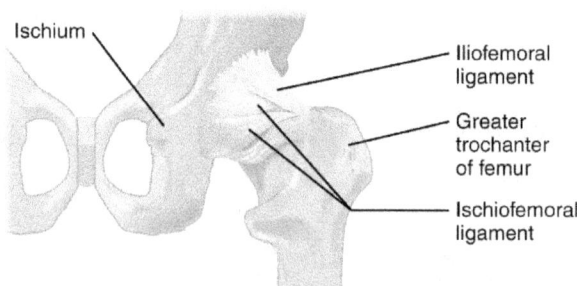

(c) Posterior view of right hip joint, capsule in place

Figure 2-3 *Right hip joint*

The hip joint facilitates six fundamental movements, aided by its surrounding soft tissues, contributing to mobility & stability of this joint.

The six hip joint motions are:

1. Flexion: Bending the hip to bring the thigh closer to the chest.
2. Extension: Straightening the hip.
3. Abduction: Moving the leg away from the body's midline.
4. Adduction: Bringing the leg back toward the body's midline.
5. Internal Rotation: Rotating of the thigh inward.
6. External Rotation: Rotating the thigh outward.

Chapter 2 - The Hip Joint

Each of these movements involves the interaction between the femur and the pelvis within various anatomical planes, as outlined in Table 2-1.

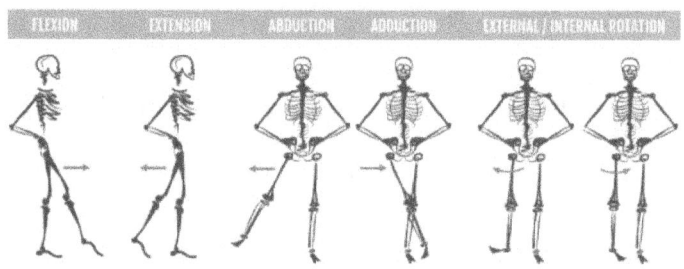

Figure 2-4 *Possible hip movements*

Following a total hip replacement surgery, patients typically aim to regain the ability to perform all these motions with the greatest possible range of motion, a goal they work towards by participating in physiotherapy sessions and maintaining a regimen of regular exercise.

The Pelvis

The pelvis stands out as the body's largest and most robust bone, forming an integral part of the hip joint.

It comprises two symmetrical halves, with each side composed of three distinct bones: the ilium, the ischium, and the pubis. Other notable features of the pelvis are:

- Obturator Foramen: This is a distinctive hollow area located below the acetabulum, through which the obturator nerve, artery, and veins traverse.

Chapter 2 - The Hip Joint

- Ischial Tuberosity: Commonly referred to as the "sitting bone," the ischial tuberosity represents the lower part of the pelvis and plays a crucial role in weight distribution when seated.

- Greater Sciatic Notch: This is a channel that accommodates the passage of the sciatic nerve, facilitating its movement through the pelvis.

These anatomical landmarks on the pelvis contribute to its unique structure and function in the context of the hip joint.

The ilium, ischium, and pubis combine to form the acetabulum, a crucial component of the hip joint situated within the pelvis.

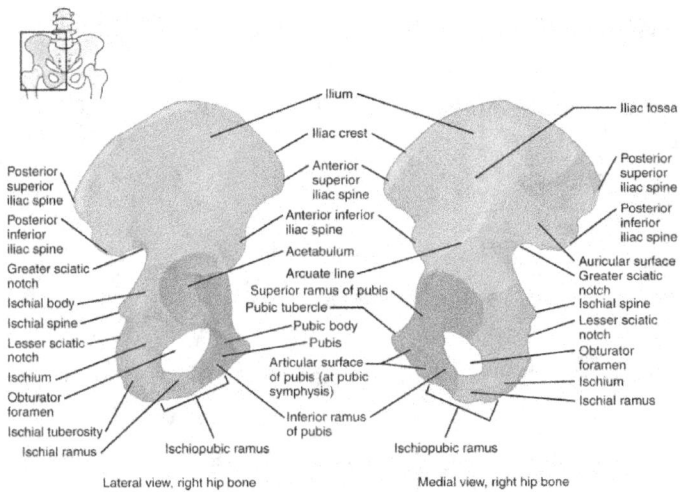

Figure 2-5 *The pelvis bone, lateral (left) and medial (right) view*

The acetabulum takes on a deep, cup-like structure that envelops the head of the femur at the hip joint.

Joint stability is maintained through the collaborative efforts of the joint capsule, the iliofemoral and pubofemoral ligaments, and the

Chapter 2 - The Hip Joint

ligamentum teres, all of which work together to secure the head of the femur within the acetabulum.

In total hip replacement surgery, these ligaments, including the joint capsule and the ligamentum teres, are typically removed and replaced with hip implant components. This process contributes to the occurrence of hip replacement dislocations following surgery.

A typical situation highlighting the potential risk of hip joint dislocation occurs when an individual with a hip implant is seated on the toilet and attempts to retrieve an item from the floor, such as pulling up their trousers from the ground or picking up a toilet roll.

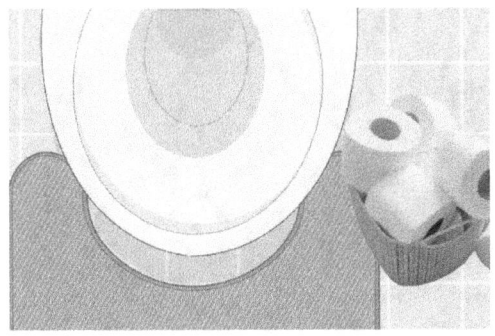

Figure 2-6 *Keep essential items at reach*

In the above scenario, as the individual bends down, they may experience a sudden pop, indicating hip joint dislocation. In such cases, immediate medical attention and revision surgery may be required.

Therefore, it is of paramount importance for joint replacement patients to follow the advice provided by the medical team about post-surgery protocols & restrictions.

The Femur

The femur stands as the longest bone in the human body. Our focus here centres on the proximal end of the femur, which forms a vital part of the hip joint. Notably, the head of the femur is not a perfect sphere; it features a small, cup-like depression known as the fovea or fovea capitis, which connects to the ligamentum teres.

One key aspect of the hip joint is the angle of inclination. This term refers to the angle in the frontal plane, formed between the femoral neck and the femur's shaft.

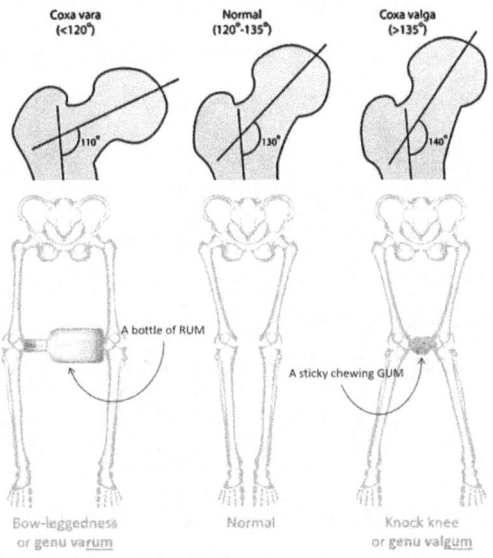

Figure 2-7 *The angle of inclination's impact on the knee joint alignment*

Typically, the angle of inclination measures approximately 125 degrees in individuals with a well-aligned standing posture. This specific angle plays a crucial role in aligning the hip and knee joints so that the knee joint effectively supports the body's weight.

Hip Implants

Total hip replacement (THR or THA) encompasses a diverse range of products available on the market, tailored to various purposes and stages of hip replacement.

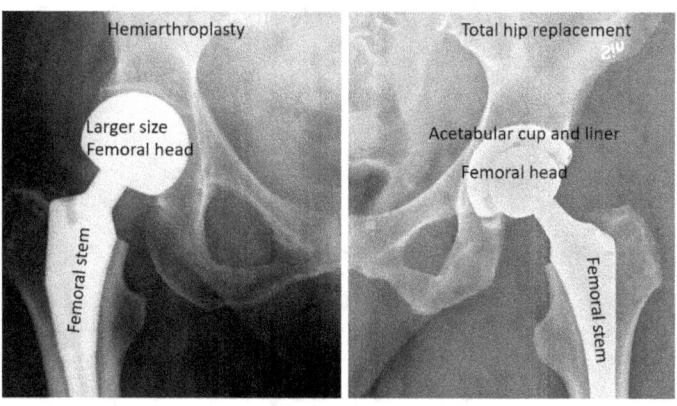

Figure 2-8 *Left: hemiarthroplasty, right: total hip replacement*

Traditionally, hip replacements are categorised into two primary types: total hip replacement and hemi hip replacement, employed in hemiarthroplasty procedures.

Total hip replacement comprises four key components:

1. Mono-Block or Modular Femoral Stem: This metal component is inserted into the femoral shaft to serve as an anchor.

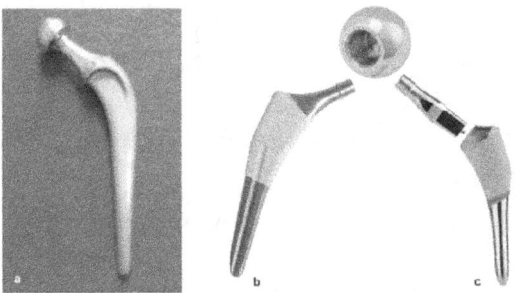

Figure 2-9 *Monoblock (a), vs modular (b, c) hip system (by Irena Gotman)*

Chapter 2 - The Hip Joint

2. Head of the Implant: Made from metal or ceramic, this component attaches to the tip of the metal stem.

3. Ceramic or Polymer Liner: Providing a smooth articulation surface within the joint, this liner enhances joint function.

4. Metal Acetabular Cup or Shell: Fixed within the acetabulum, this component forms the socket portion of the hip joint.

Conversely, hemi hip replacement or partial hip replacement (used in hemiarthroplasty) differs in that it lacks the acetabular cup or shell component. Instead, the head of the implant articulates directly within the natural acetabulum.

Hemiarthroplasty is typically performed when the surgeon determines that the bone and cartilage inside the acetabulum are of sufficient quality to function effectively in combination with the artificial head and stem.

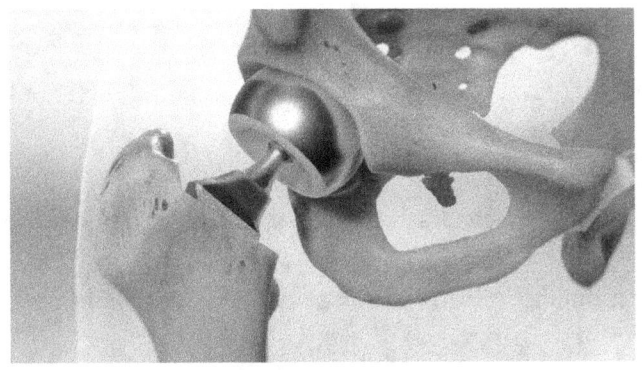

Figure 2-10 *Hemiarthroplasty*

This approach is commonly employed in cases involving a fractured neck of the femur, rather than for joint replacement to alleviate pain and inflammation resulting from arthritis.

In such a case, the damaged femoral head is removed and replaced with a prosthetic femoral head, which may be metal or ceramic.

Hemi hip replacement may provide pain relief and improved function, but it may not be suitable for long-term use in patients with pre-existing hip joint conditions.

Finally, there is hip joint resurfacing. Hip resurfacing is a surgical option that preserves more of the patient's natural bone compared to a total hip replacement.

In a hip resurfacing procedure, the damaged surface of the femoral head is reshaped and capped with a metal prosthesis, while the acetabulum may or may not be replaced.

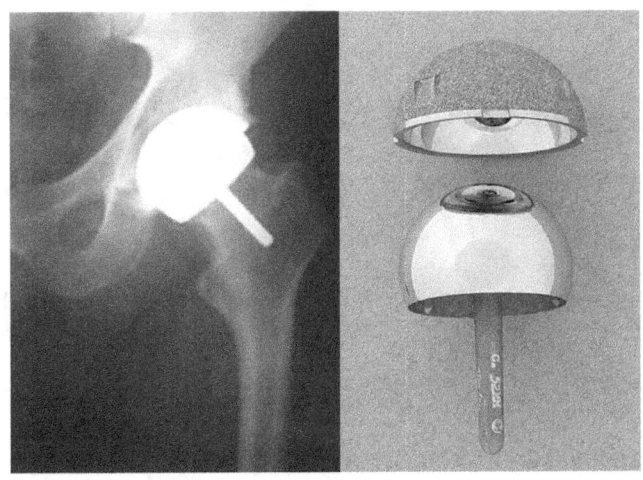

Figure 2-11 *Metal-on-metal hip resurfacing system - "M-o-M" means that both the joint's ball and socket components are made of metal*

This approach is often chosen for younger, active patients with good bone quality, as it may provide more durability and easier revision options in the future.

Femoral Component or Stem

A femoral stem possesses two key distinguishable attributes: the taper and the fixation surface.

The optimal design of a stem aims to efficiently transmit both torsional and axial loads to the bone while minimising the generation of damaging peak stresses and preventing excessive micro-movement.

Contemporary stem designs prioritise long-term mechanical stability, even when subjected to repetitive loading.

Several features of the stem's shape significantly impact the in vivo behaviour of femoral components.

Overall Shape:

This can be either straight or anatomical, tailored to the specific needs of the patient.

Cross-Section Shape:

It may take on various cross-section forms, such as oval or square, influencing the stem's mechanical properties.

Presence of a Collar:

Some stems include a collar, which can affect how the implant interacts with the surrounding bone.

Chapter 2 - The Hip Joint

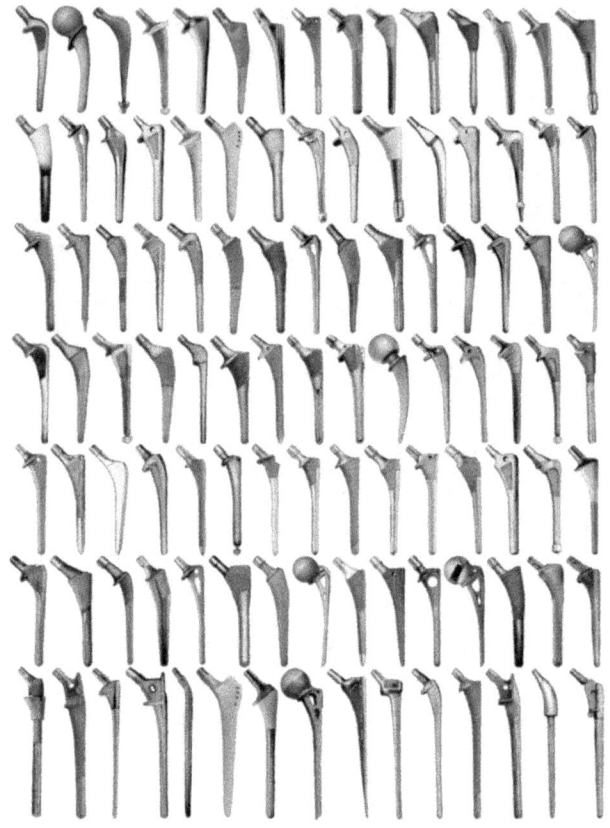

Figure 2-12 *The above poster published in 2003, courtesy of Annie Gallup, is the display of 105 various designs of modular and mono-block THA femoral components*

Shape & Size of the Proximal Tip or Trunnion:

The trunnion or male taper of the stem may exhibit distinct shapes, sizes and angles that influence the size and positioning of the femoral head attachment.

Shape of the Distal Tip:

The tip of the stem may exhibit distinct shapes that influence its positioning within the femur.

Stem Length:

The length is an important consideration, as it determines how deeply it is inserted into the femur.

Edge Roundness:

The degree to which the edges of the stem are rounded can impact its performance and stability.

Properly rounded edges promote even stress distribution, smoother movement, and overall better long-term performance of the hip replacement

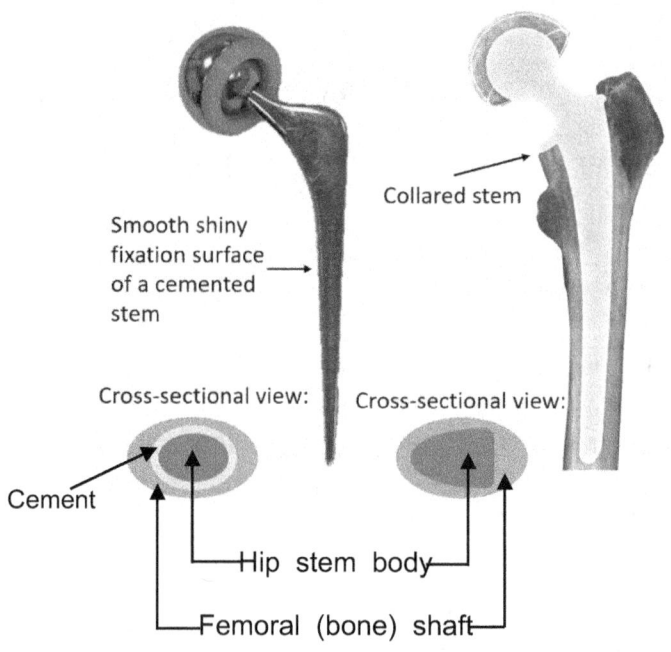

Figure 2-13 *Two examples of femoral component designs (there are several other designs available on the market)*

Stem Material and Surface Finish

All these features collectively contribute to the behaviour and performance of femoral components in the body.

Femoral stems are typically crafted from materials such as titanium and medical grade stainless steel which are biocompatible.

This quality ensures that none of these metal alloys have any adverse effects on the human body. These materials are favoured for their advantageous combination of strength, corrosion resistance, and wear resistance, making them the primary choices for implant materials.

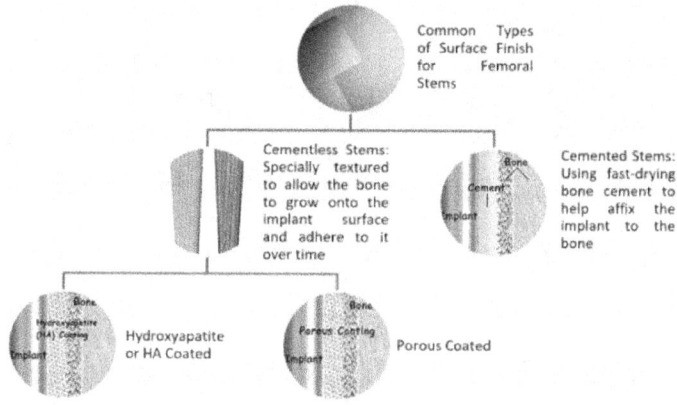

Figure 2-14 *Common types of surface finish for femoral stems*

In the late 1970s, coatings (e.g. porous coating) were introduced to enhance the surface properties of implants, aiming to improve the process of osseointegration. Subsequent research and advancements in manufacturing techniques resulted in better clinical outcomes.

Various methods are employed to create porous metallic coatings, including sintering, electron beam deposition, thermal spraying, and plasma spraying. Another coating used on implants' surfaces is a white powder-like substance called hydroxyapatite.

One common method for depositing hydroxyapatite (HA) is through the plasma spray technique. This process is carried out at high temperatures, typically around 15,000°C, and under a vacuum. HA particles are projected onto the metallic material at a rapid speed of 300 meters per second.

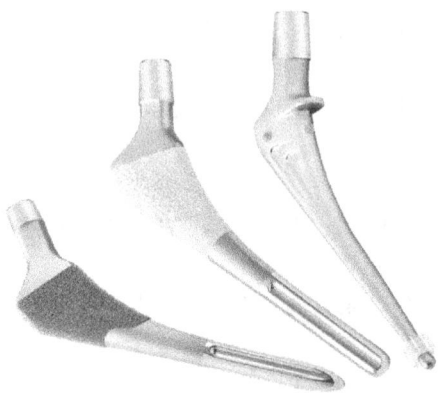

Figure 2-15 *Hip system, porous coating (left), HA coating (middle) and smooth surface finish (right)*

The metallic substrate is intentionally roughened to facilitate the adhesion of bone cells to the implant surface. This combination of techniques and materials has significantly contributed to the success of orthopaedic implants.

A cemented stem is a versatile choice for orthopaedic situations, suitable even when there is a femoral deformity.

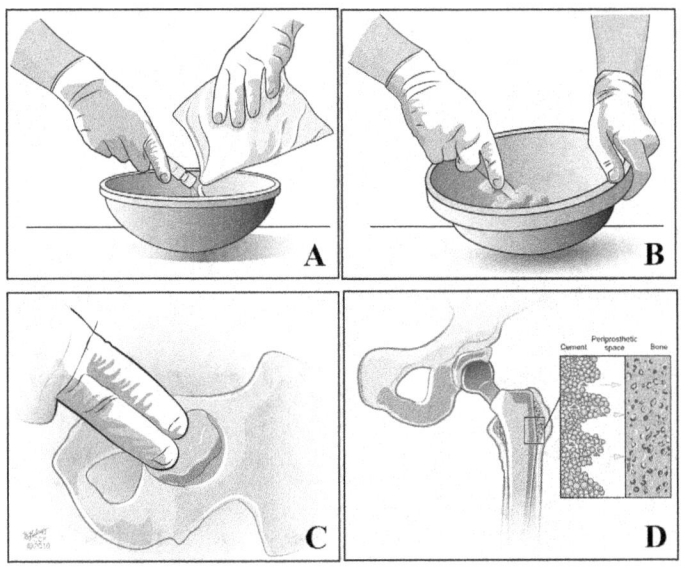

Figure 2-16 *Cement application (by V Athans)*

The use of "bone cement" allows for precise positioning of implant components in alignment with the patient's anatomy and leg length. Bone cement, also commonly known as PMMA (Polymethylmethacrylate) is typically employed for this purpose.

Femoral Head

In the context of hip replacement, the femoral head exhibits two primary features: the taper and the bearing surface. The taper represents the connection point between the head and the neck of the femoral component, while the bearing surface interacts within the acetabular liner.

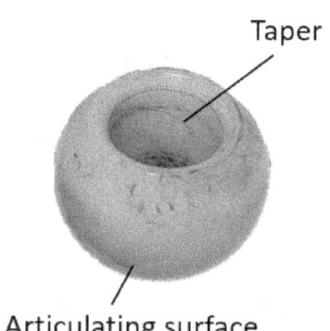

Figure 2-17 *A retrieved modular femoral head made of Alumina ceramic*

Both the material selection and the design of the femoral head should be geared toward ensuring sufficient mechanical resistance against the tensile stresses that occur along the taper junction. This consideration is crucial for the overall durability and performance of the hip implant.

The ideal size for the femoral head bearing should strike a balance between achieving the highest stability and optimal hip function while minimising wear, thus extending the longevity of total hip arthroplasty (THA).

Femoral head sizes typically range from 22 to 54 millimetres, and custom implant manufacturing allows for the production of both smaller and larger heads to suit individual patient needs.

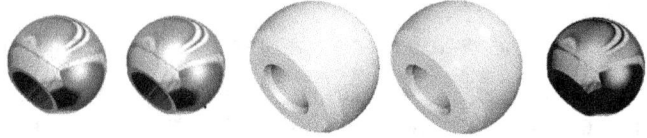

Figure 2-18 *From left to right: stainless steel, Co-Cr, Alumina ceramic, Zirconia ceramic and Oxinium™ modular femoral heads*

Femoral heads are typically crafted from either metallic or ceramic materials. The most commonly used materials for femoral heads include Cobalt-Chromium alloys, medical grade stainless steel, ceramics like alumina, zirconia and Oxinium™.

These materials are selected based on their suitability for the specific application, taking into account factors such as durability and biocompatibility.

Head Options

Modular femoral head implants are predominantly used in contemporary hip arthroplasty. The term "modular" is defined by the Cambridge Dictionary as "consisting of separate parts that, when combined, form a complete whole."

Whenever you encounter a femoral head, whether it's made of metal or ceramic, as a separate. standalone component, you are dealing with a modular head. The market offers several common types of femoral heads, including unipolar, bipolar, and dual mobility (DM) heads.

Chapter 2 - The Hip Joint

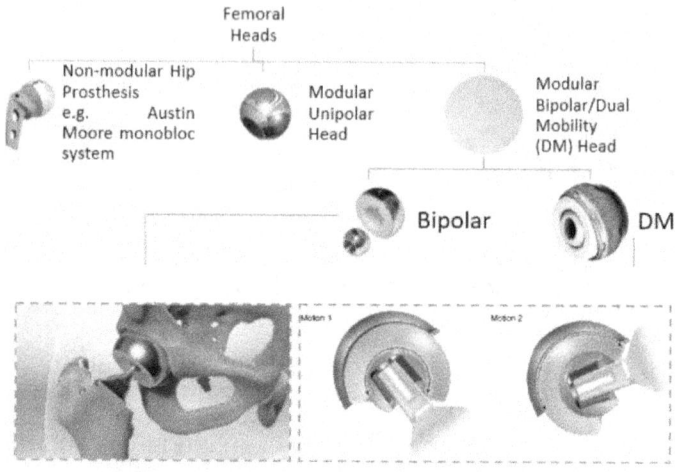

Figure 2-19 *Femoral head options*

Note, the majority of hip replacement heads you encounter are the traditional unipolar type. In the unipolar design, hip movement occurs as the femoral head articulates within the liner.

The liner is firmly fixed in position within the metal shell, and it must not exhibit any movement relative to the acetabular shell.

In the unipolar design, any movement of the liner indicates a failure of the hip implant due to liner disassociation. In such cases, a revision surgery would be necessary to replace the disassociated liner with a new one.

Bipolar hip replacement is a type of hip arthroplasty that can be used in both hemiarthroplasty and total hip arthroplasty (THA) procedures.

In bipolar hip replacement, there are two metal components: the inner femoral head and the outer acetabular component. Between them, there is a polyethylene (PE) liner.

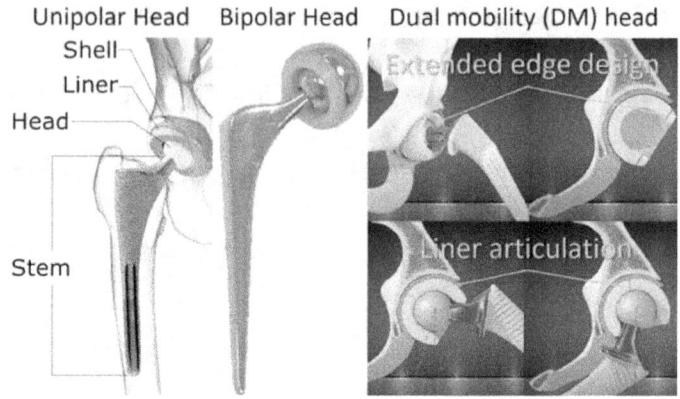

Figure 2-20 *Three designs for femoral heads: unipolar, bipolar, and dual mobility*

In hemiarthroplasty, the smaller metal head articulates inside the larger metal head, and the larger metal head articulates directly within the acetabulum (hip socket).

This design is often used when only the femoral side of the hip joint needs to be replaced, such as in cases of femoral neck fractures.

Whereas in THA, the bipolar design is used similarly to the hemiarthroplasty setup, with the larger metal head articulating within a liner fixed inside the acetabular shell.

The primary advantage of bipolar hip replacement is that it can potentially reduce the risk of dislocation, especially in cases where the hip socket (acetabulum) is not damaged.

Dual mobility hip replacement is primarily used in total hip arthroplasty (THA) procedures. In this design, the femoral head snaps into the polyethylene (PE) liner, and both the head and liner can articulate and provide motion in the hip joint. This design allows for greater mobility and flexibility.

The reason behind developing dual mobility system is to reduce the risk of dislocation by providing multiple points of articulation within the hip joint, enhancing stability. However, it's important to note that while dual mobility implants are believed to reduce dislocation rates, there is still limited conclusive evidence supporting this claim.

Dual mobility hip replacements are typically used in THA cases where both the femoral and acetabular sides of the hip joint require replacement. This means dual mobility heads are not suitable nor recommended for "hemiarthroplasty" surgical operation.

Acetabular Liner

The acetabular liner is a critical component placed inside the hip joint during total hip replacement surgery. Its primary purpose is to enhance stability and provide a smooth surface for articulation within the replaced hip joint.

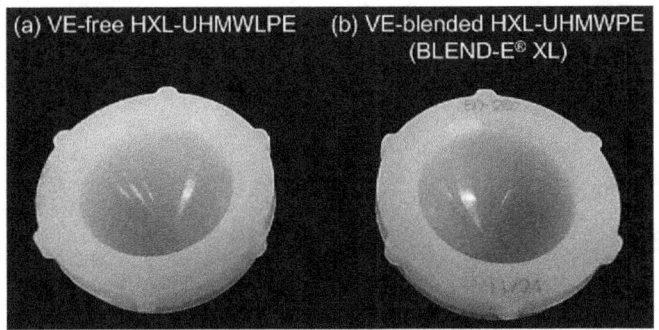

Figure 2-21 *Liners (a) HXL-UHMWPE, (b) Vitamin E-blended HXL-UHMWPE (by Yasuhito Takahashi)*

Liner Material

Acetabular liners are typically made from various materials, and the choice of material can impact the performance of the hip replacement. The most common materials for acetabular liners are:

- Polyethylene (PE) - This can include ultra-high molecular weight polyethylene (UHMWPE) or cross-linked UHMWPE (XLPE). These are the most frequently used materials for liners. There's also PEEK (or polyetheretherketone), and vitamin-E infused or blended highly-XLPE.

- Ceramic - Ceramic liners are an alternative option, offering their own set of advantages and disadvantages.

- Metal - While metal liners were used in the past, they have become less common and are now being withdrawn from the market due to concerns about metal-on-metal hip replacements.

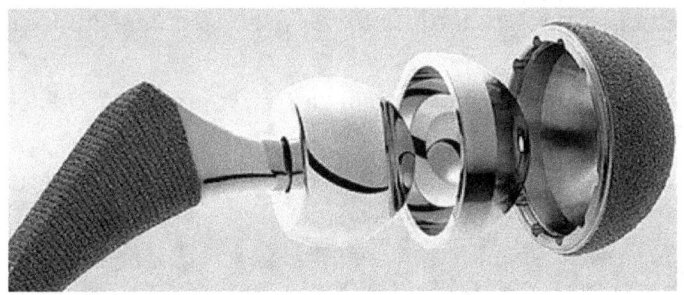

Figure 2-22 *Metal stem head, liner & cup making a M-o-M bearing which is no longer on the market (By Gregory A. Tocks, D.O.)*

Head-Liner Combinations

Now that you have a better understanding of the femoral head and liner components, let's explore the part of the hip joint that allows it to move, known as the hip joint "bearing".

Depending on the material used for the femoral head and the acetabular liner, various head-liner combinations are possible. Each combination has its own unique advantages and disadvantages. Some common head-liner combinations include:

- Ceramic-on-polyethylene (CoP)
- Ceramic-on-ceramic (CoC)
- Metal-on-polyethylene (MoP)

- Metal-on-metal[2] (MoM)

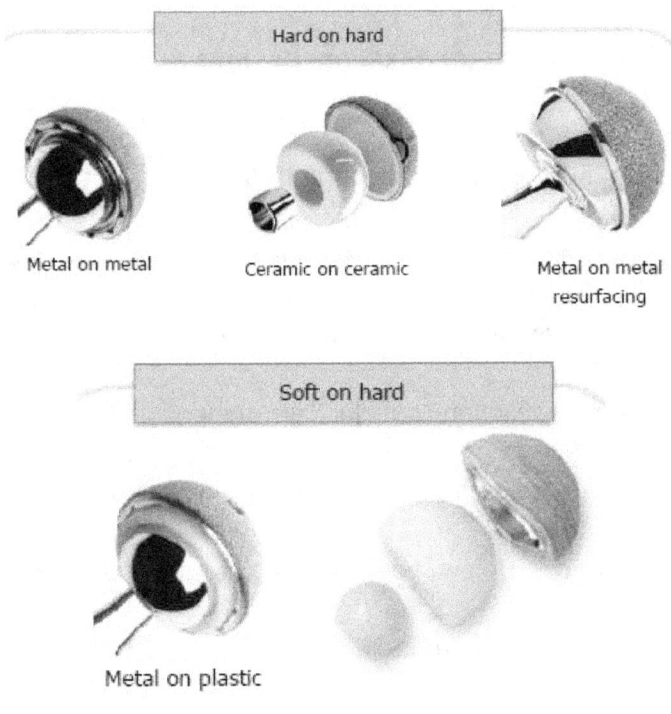

Figure 2-23 *Head-liner combination examples*

---

[2] Note, M-o-M implants have faced concerns related to potential wear, metal ion release, and adverse reactions in some patients, leading to their decreased use in favour of alternative materials like ceramic or polyethylene.

Chapter 2 - The Hip Joint

Liner Locking or Fixation Designs

Liner fixation is an important aspect of total hip replacement, and different fixation systems are used to secure the acetabular liner in place. The choice of fixation design can depend on factors such as the type of liner used and the surgeon's preference. Below you can see what's commonly available on the market.

- Press-Fit Liners - These liners are designed to fit tightly into the acetabular component or cup without the need for additional fixation mechanisms. The press-fit design relies on the interference fit between the liner and the cup to hold it in place.

- Locking Ring - Locking rings are often used in conjunction with constrained liners. These rings help secure the liner in place and prevent dislocation of the hip joint.

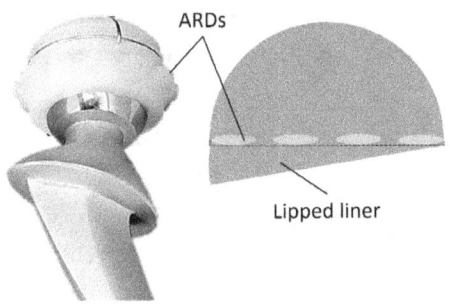

Figure 2-24 *Liner fixation examples, anti-rotation device (ARD) design & lipped or elevated design*

- Anti-Rotation Device (ARD) Scallop Design - Some acetabular shell designs incorporate multiple Anti-Rotation Device (ARD) scallops that accept ARD tabs on the polyethylene liner. This design enhances stability by preventing liner rotation within the shell.

- Lipped or Elevated Liner Design - In this design, the acetabular liner has an asymmetrical shape with a lip or elevated edge. This feature can provide additional stability by helping to hold the liner and head in place.

- Cemented Liners - In some cases, the polyethylene liner may be cemented directly into the acetabulum using bone cement. This method provides strong fixation and stability. No metal shell would be used in this method.

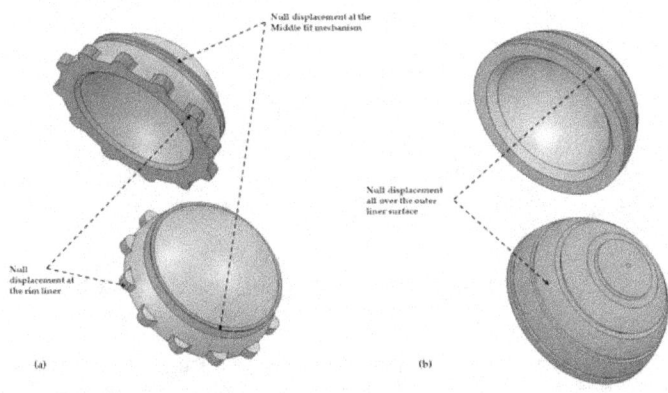

Figure 2-25 *Left: uncemented (ARD) design, right: cemented liner design (by Loreto Barrios)*

The choice of liner fixation design is determined by factors such as the specific type of liner being used, the patient's anatomy, and the surgeon's preference. Surgeons aim to select the fixation system that will provide the best stability and longevity for the hip replacement while minimising the risk of complications like dislocation.

Acetabular Shell

While the terms "acetabular cup" and "acetabular shell" can sometimes be used interchangeably, they are often used to describe slightly different configurations within the total hip replacement modular system.

The acetabular cup can function on its own as the socket, but when used with a liner (typically ceramic or polyethylene), it is referred to as an acetabular shell.

The acetabular shell accommodates the liner and provides a smooth surface for the head of the femoral component to articulate, allowing for motion in the hip joint.

Variety of Shapes and Sizes

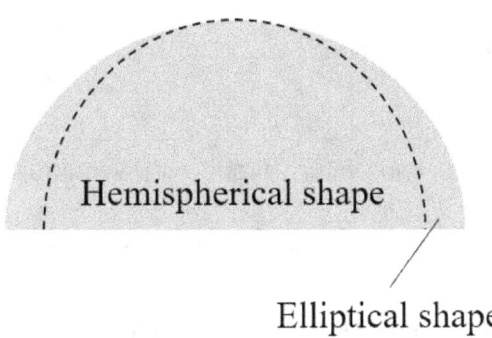

Figure 2-26 *Hemispherical vs elliptical shell designs (exaggerated for visibility)*

Acetabular shells or cups come in various shapes and sizes to accommodate the specific needs of each patient. The most common designs are hemispherical and elliptical cups.

Hemispherical cups have a rounded shape similar to half of a sphere, while elliptical cups have a slightly flared or elongated shape resembling an ellipse.

Cup Fixation Options

There are two main types of acetabular shell fixation options, cemented and cementless. Cemented cups are fixed in place using bone cement, providing immediate stability.

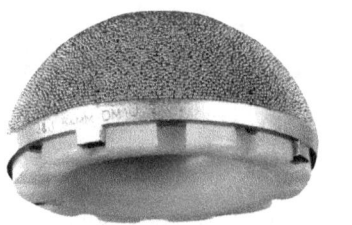 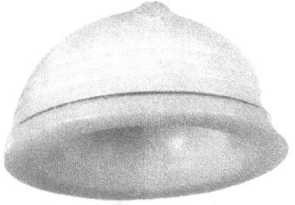

Figure 2-27 *Left: a cementless acetabular shell, right: a cemented acetabular cup (by D.S.Angadi)*

In contrast, cementless cups rely on bone ingrowth for long-term fixation.

Before implantation, the acetabulum is prepared to create a bed of vascular cancellous bone, which encourages the natural bone to grow into and secure the acetabular component in place.

The choice between cemented and cementless acetabular shells depends on factors such as the patient's bone quality, surgeon preference, and the specific requirements of the hip replacement procedure.

The goal is to achieve a stable and durable fixation that allows long-term function & success.

Acetabular Component Material and Coating

The acetabular shell has two critical surfaces. The fixation surface & the taper. The fixation surface is often coated with hydroxyapatite or a porous metal coating to promote bone ingrowth (sometimes with screw holes to enable screw-fixation to acetabulum), ensuring secure fixation.

The taper provides a smooth surface where a polyethylene or ceramic liner attaches, allowing the head of the femoral component to articulate smoothly within the hip joint (on the liner bearing surface).

Primary vs. Revision Hip Implants

In the context of hip replacement surgery, there are two main categories: primary and revision hip implants. Primary surgery involves using a hip implant to replace a diseased or worn-out hip joint.

It is the first joint replacement procedure performed on a patient, addressing an injured or diseased joint.

Revision surgery is performed when a previously implanted hip implant is no longer functioning properly or has complications.

Chapter 2 - The Hip Joint

A patient can undergo up to a maximum of two primary hip replacement procedures, one for each hip.

Any subsequent operations on the same hip(s) are referred to as revision surgery, such as first revision surgery, second revision surgery, and so on.

Revision surgery is necessary when there is a need to replace, repair, or modify a previously implanted hip prosthesis due to issues like implant wear, instability, loosening, infection, or other complications.

Revision surgery for hip replacement is indeed more complex & challenging than primary hip .

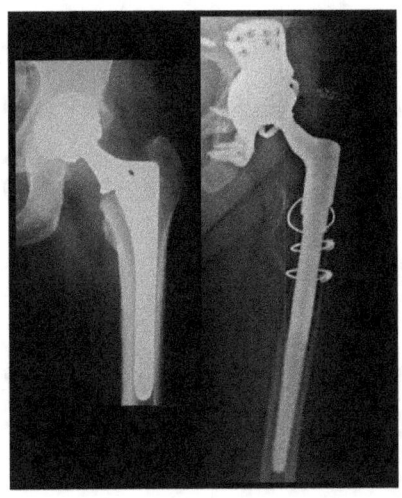

Figure 2-28 *Left: a primary total hip replacement, right: a revision total hip replacement. Note the difference in the size and shape of the parts*

The key considerations in revision surgery include simplifying the procedure and effectively managing femoral bone loss, whether it existed prior to revision or occurred during the revision operation.

Note, streamlining the revision surgery process is crucial to achieve successful outcomes. Surgeons aim to simplify the procedure while addressing any complications or issues related to the existing implant.

Managing bone loss in the femur is a critical aspect of revision surgery. Surgeons must address any bone loss, which can result from various factors, including implant loosening or bone resorption. Different techniques and implant options may be used to address bone loss effectively.

Knowing the specifics of the primary implant used in the initial hip replacement is essential for successful revision surgery. Surgeons typically identify the manufacturer and model of the implant by reviewing the patient's medical records or examining radiographic images of the implant. This information guides the selection of compatible revision components.

Radiographic images, such as X-rays or other imaging studies, are valuable tools in identifying the primary implant and assessing its condition. These images help the surgeon plan the revision surgery and determine the appropriate components needed for the new implant.

Patient medical records provide essential information about the type of implant used, the date of the primary surgery, and any relevant details about the patient's medical history. Reviewing these records is an integral part of the pre-operative assessment for revision surgery.

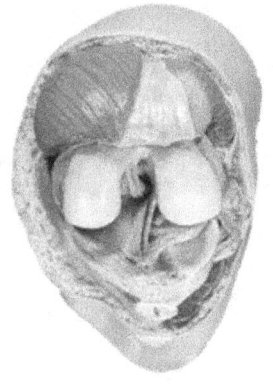
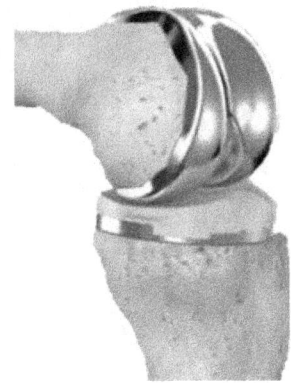

Chapter 3

The Knee Joint

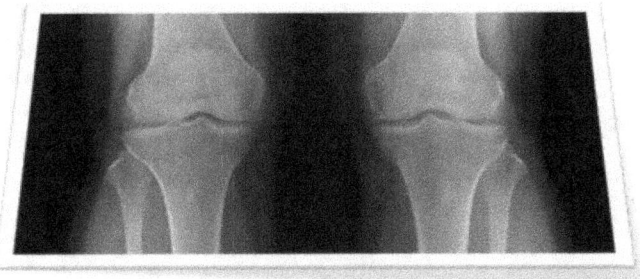

Chapter 3 - The Knee Joint

An Introduction to the Knee Joint

In order to grasp the content of this section more effectively, it is essential to have a good understanding of the knee joint's intricate nature. This chapter offers a concise introduction to the key attributes and operations of the knee joint.

To enhance your comprehension, it is highly recommend that you study the reference anatomical planes & motion axes in chapter two.

The distal femur and proximal tibia are two major bones that come together to form the knee joint.

The distal femur refers to the lower part of the femur bone, which is the thigh bone, situated closer to the knee joint.

It consists of two rounded condyles, the medial condyle on the inner side, and the lateral condyle on the outer side. These condyles articulate with the corresponding structures on the proximal tibia, allowing for the flexion & extension movements.

The proximal tibia is the upper part of the tibia , which is one of the two lower leg bones. It features a flat upper surface with two prominent plateaus, the medial & the lateral plateau.

The proximal tibia plays a crucial role in supporting and stabilising the knee joint.

Chapter 3 - The Knee Joint

The distal femur and proximal tibia come together at the knee joint, forming a synovial hinge joint.

Articular cartilage covers the surfaces of the femoral condyles and tibial plateaus, providing a smooth, low -friction surface for movement.

The distal femur and proximal tibia work in concert, allowing for the essential functions of the knee joint, including flexion, extension, and limited rotation.

This structural and functional integration is vital for the overall stability and mobility of the knee, supporting activities such as walking, running, and weight-bearing.

Anatomy and Biomechanics of the Knee Joint

One of the body's most extensive and complex joints is the knee, composed of two primary combinations: the tibiofemoral joint (this is what we often refer to as "the knee joint") and the patellofemoral joint.

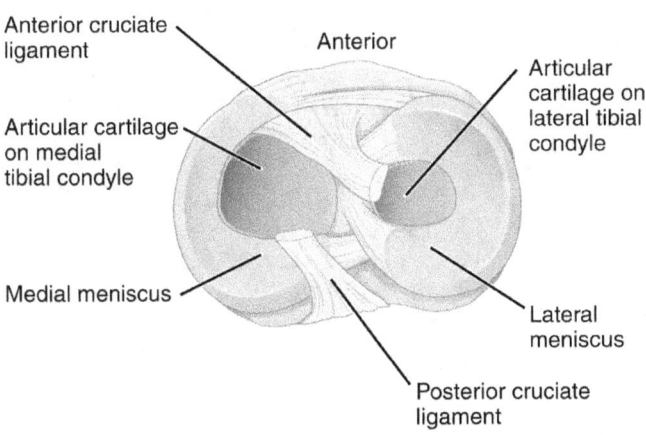

Figure 3-1 *Right tibia superior (CC BY-SA-NC)*

Chapter 3 - The Knee Joint

The patellofemoral joint (PFJ) forms when the patella interacts with the distal femur. The knee joint enables various movements, including flexion, extension, and to a limited degree, medial and lateral rotation.

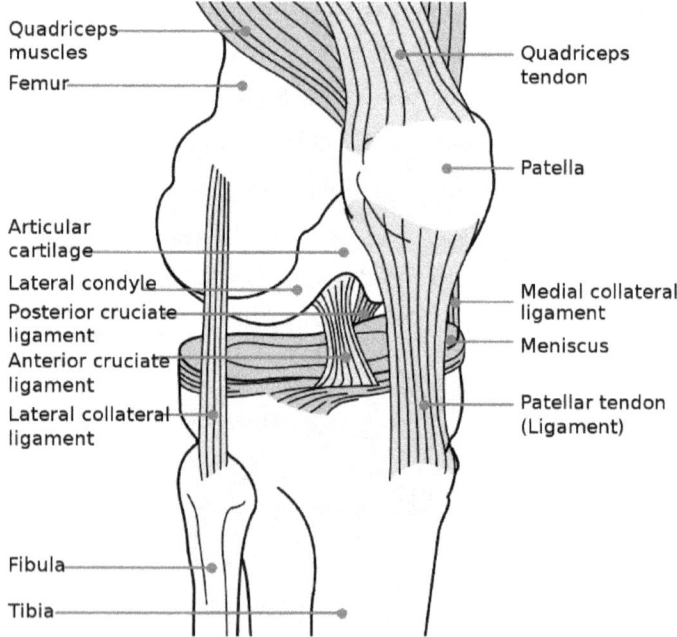

Figure 3-2 *Knee joint anterolateral (CC BY-SA)*

As described in Chapter two, the angle of inclination in the hip refers to the angle formed between the femoral neck and the shaft of the femur.

This angle is measured in the frontal plane of the body. It's a key anatomical feature because it determines the orientation of the femur as it connects to the hip joint.

When the proximal femur has an angle of inclination of 125 degrees, it directs the shaft of the femur toward the midline of the body. In other words, the femur is oriented in such a way that it points slightly inward toward the centre of the body.

Chapter 3 - The Knee Joint

The femur, with its angle of inclination, eventually articulates with the tibia at the knee joint. The way the femur connects to the tibia is crucial for proper knee function.

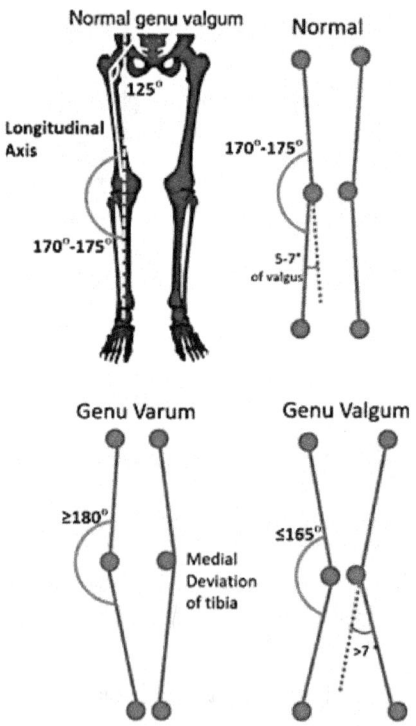

Figure 3-3 *Frontal plane deviations of the knee, top: normal, bottom: varus & valgus alignment*

The lateral knee angle is the angle formed between the femur and the tibia when looking at the knee joint from the front of the body. In a typical, healthy alignment, the femur aligns with the tibia to create a lateral knee angle ranging from 170 to 175 degrees.

Remember, a proper angle of inclination ensures that the femur and tibia align correctly. When the femur's inclination directs its shaft toward the midline, it allows for a natural alignment with the tibia.

This alignment is essential for distributing forces and loads properly across the knee joint during activities like walking, running, and standing. It

Chapter 3 - The Knee Joint

helps prevent undue stress or strain on the knee structures.

The lateral knee angle of 170 to 175 degrees indicates that the femur projects slightly outward or laterally in relation to the tibia. This alignment contributes to the stability and proper function of the knee joint, as it helps to resist excessive lateral forces and maintains joint integrity.

Therefore, the angle of inclination in the hip is a critical factor in ensuring the proper alignment of the femur with the tibia at the knee joint. This alignment, in turn, influences the lateral knee angle, which is important for knee stability and function.

It's important to also remember that the lateral knee angle, typically ranges from 170 to 175 degrees, indicating that the femur is only slightly laterally offset from the tibia. This is one of the considerations in any knee replacement surgical operation.

"Genu varum" and "genu valgum" are terms used to describe two different knee deformities based on the alignment of the knee joint and can affect the way the knees are positioned relative to each other and to the rest of the body.

Genu varum, also known as "bowleg," is a condition where the knees are abnormally spaced apart from each other when the person is standing with their feet together. This results in a

Chapter 3 - The Knee Joint

visible gap between the knees, resembling the shape of a bow (hence the name "bowleg").

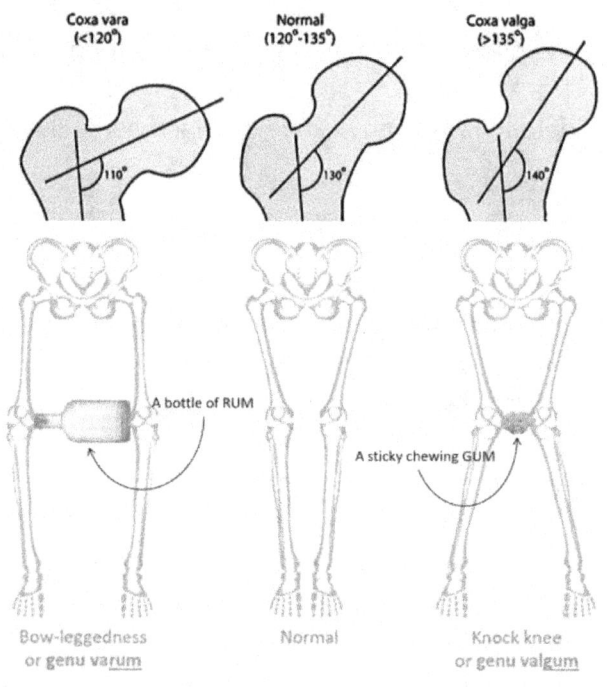

Figure 3-4 *"Genu varum" vs. "genu valgum"*

Genu varum can be caused by various factors, including genetics, metabolic disorders, or developmental issues. In children, it can be a normal developmental stage that typically corrects itself as the child grows.

Severe genu varum can affect the alignment of the entire lower limb, potentially leading to joint pain, instability, and abnormal gait patterns.

Genu valgum, also known as "knock-knee," is a condition where the knees are abnormally close together when the person is standing with their feet apart. In this condition, the knees appear to angle inward, often causing the ankles to touch each other while the knees are apart.

Genu valgum can also have various causes, including genetics, developmental factors, or underlying medical conditions. It can occur in childhood but may persist into adulthood if not corrected.

Like genu varum, severe genu valgum can affect the alignment of the lower limbs, potentially leading to joint pain, instability, and an abnormal gait.

Both genu varum and genu valgum can be assessed and diagnosed by orthopaedic specialists through physical examination and imaging studies like X-rays.

Treatment options may include physical therapy, orthotic devices, or in severe cases, surgical interventions to correct the alignment.

It's important to note that mild variations in knee alignment are common and not necessarily indicative of a medical problem.

However, persistent or severe deformities may warrant medical evaluation and treatment, especially if they lead to discomfort, pain, or difficulty with daily activities.

The next concept that goes hand-in-hand with alignment is "overcorrecting in joint replacement", specifically in the context of total knee replacement (TKR).

Overcorrection refers to a situation where the surgeon makes an adjustment to the alignment of the knee joint that goes beyond the optimal or natural alignment of the patient's knee.

Overcorrection can lead to several problems and complications. This is because human knee joint is designed to function within a certain range of angles and alignments.

Overcorrecting by making the knee joint either too straight (genu varum) or too bent (genu valgum) can disrupt the natural biomechanics of the knee.

This can result in abnormal stress distribution on the joint surfaces, leading to accelerated wear and tear of the artificial joint components.

Overcorrection can lead to instability in the replaced knee.

For instance, if the knee is over-straightened (genu varum), it may become more difficult for the patient to fully extend the leg.

Conversely, if it's over-bent (genu valgum), it can become unstable during walking or standing. This instability can increase the risk of falls and injury. An overcorrected knee can limit the patient's range of motion.

If the knee is excessively straight, it can impede the patient's ability to bend the knee fully, affecting their ability to perform everyday activities like sitting, kneeling, or climbing stairs.

Chapter 3 - The Knee Joint

Conversely, an over-bent knee can restrict full extension, leading to problems with walking/gait.

Overcorrection can cause increased pain and discomfort in the replaced knee. The unnatural alignment can put additional stress on the soft tissues surrounding the joint, leading to pain, swelling, and inflammation.

The artificial components used in total knee replacement are designed to function optimally within a certain range of alignment.

Over time, overcorrection can cause premature wear and loosening of these components, leading to the need for revision surgery to correct the alignment and replace damaged components.

Ultimately, overcorrection can result in suboptimal functional outcomes for the patient. The goal of TKR is to restore the knee's function and alleviate pain.

Overcorrection can hinder the achievement of these goals, leading to dissatisfaction with the surgical outcome.

To avoid overcorrection and its associated complications, surgeons rely on pre-operative planning, precise measurements, and advanced surgical techniques.

They aim to achieve a balance between correcting the deformity that necessitated the knee replacement and maintaining the natural biomechanics of the knee joint as closely as possible.

Additionally, ongoing post-operative care, physical therapy, and monitoring are essential to ensure that the knee heals properly and functions optimally after surgery.

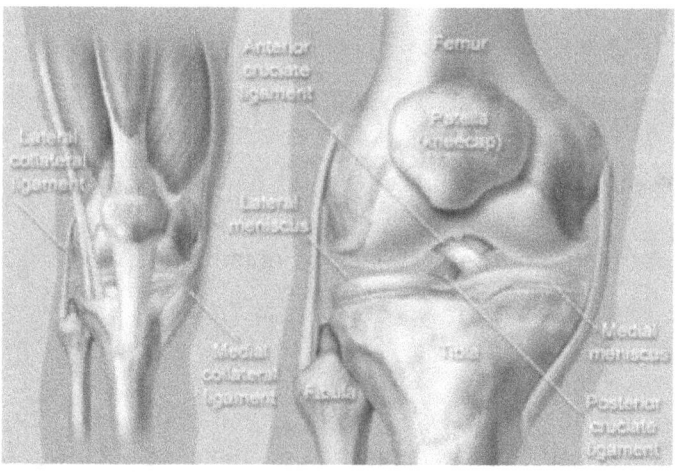

Figure 3-5 *Limited soft tissue surrounding the knee joint*

In contrast to the hip joint, the stability of the knee joint doesn't primarily rely on the congruence of the bony surfaces or their natural design at the distal femur and proximal tibia.

Instead, it heavily depends on the integrity of the soft tissues that encompass the knee joint, which includes tendons and ligaments.

Many of these soft tissues are modified or removed during total knee replacement surgery. Here are a few examples:

- The anterior cruciate ligament (ACL) serves to inhibit the posterior movement of the femur relative to the tibia (or the anterior movement of the tibia relative to the femur).

Chapter 3 - The Knee Joint

- The posterior cruciate ligament (PCL) functions to hinder the anterior movement of the femur relative to the tibia (or the posterior movement of the tibia relative to the femur).

- The medial (MCL) and lateral (LCL) collateral ligaments are responsible for restraining lateral movement of the femur, preventing it from shifting side to side.

- The medial and lateral menisci, two C-shaped pieces of cartilage, play the role of shock absorbers between the femur and tibia, cushioning and stabilising the joint.

- Numerous bursae, fluid-filled sacs, aid in facilitating smooth movement of the knee joint, reducing friction and preventing irritation between adjacent structures.

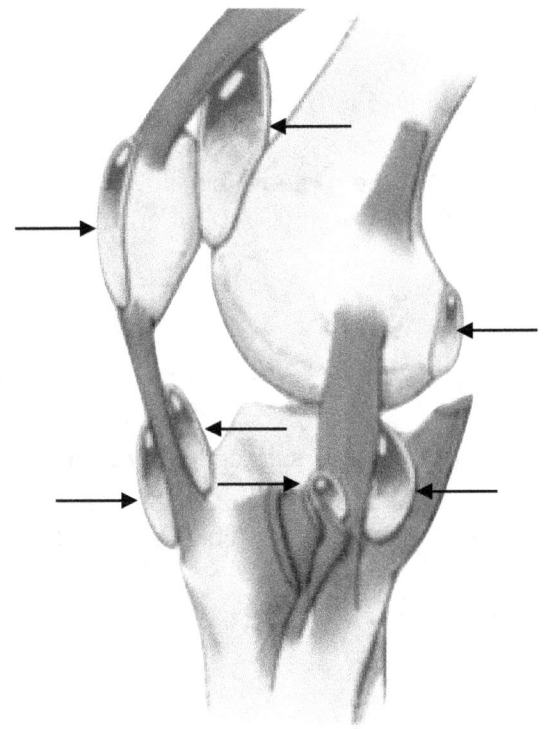

Figure 3-6 *Knee bursae highlighted by arrows*

These soft tissues collectively contribute to the complex mechanics and stability of the knee joint,

Chapter 3 - The Knee Joint

highlighting their importance in ensuring proper functioning and preventing injuries.

For example, the menisci, often referred to as the "knee cartilages" are crucial and integral components of the knee joint's structure and function.

The menisci are located on the proximal tibia, specifically on the top surface, where they serve as cushions between the tibia and the femur (thigh bone).

There are two menisci in each knee joint: the medial meniscus and the lateral meniscus. The medial meniscus is positioned on the inner side of the knee, while the lateral meniscus is on the outer side.

The medial and lateral menisci are crescent-shaped fibrocartilaginous discs, meaning they have a curved or moon-like shape.

This curved shape allows them to conform to the rounded ends of the femur and provide an additional layer of cushioning and support to the knee joint.

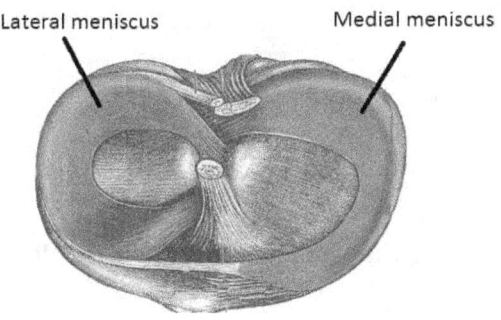

Figure 3-7 *Knee menisci*

Chapter 3 - The Knee Joint

One of the primary functions of the menisci is to distribute the load and forces placed on the knee joint.

They help to spread the weight and stress evenly across the joint, reducing the risk of excessive wear and tear on the articular cartilage (the smooth, shiny tissue covering the ends of bones) of the femur and tibia.

The menisci also contribute to knee joint stability by enhancing the fit between the femur and tibia.

They deepen the articular surfaces of the tibia, creating a better congruence with the rounded condyles of the femur, thus helping to prevent excessive sliding or shifting of the bones during movement.

When the knee experiences impact or compression, such as during running or jumping, the menisci act as shock absorbers.

They absorb and dissipate some of the forces, reducing the impact on the bones and protecting the joint from damage.

The menisci help with the lubrication and nourishment of the knee joint.

They distribute synovial fluid (a lubricating fluid found within the joint) and nutrients to the articular cartilage, which is essential for maintaining joint health.

Chapter 3 - The Knee Joint

Moreover, the knee joint's stability and range of motion are highly dependent on the intricate network of soft tissues, which include tendons, ligaments, and muscles.

These structures work together to facilitate movement while also maintaining the joint's stability.

Tendons are tough, fibrous tissues that connect muscles to bones. In the knee joint, tendons play a critical role in transmitting the force generated by muscles to move the joint.

The quadriceps tendon, for example, connects the quadriceps muscles to the patella (kneecap), and the patellar tendon further connects the patella to the tibia. These tendons are essential for extending the knee (straightening the leg).

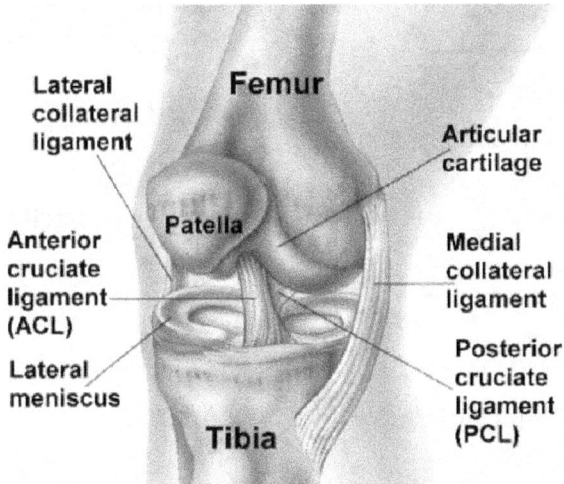

Figure 3-8 *Ligaments (by Dr Ralph Gambardella)*

Ligaments are strong bands of connective tissue that connect bone to bone. In the knee joint, various ligaments provide stability and limit excessive movement. These ligaments (ACL, PCL, MCL, LCL) work together to maintain the joint's stability during various movements.

Chapter 3 - The Knee Joint

Muscles surrounding the knee joint also play a crucial role in producing movement and controlling joint stability.

The quadriceps muscles, located on the front of the thigh, are responsible for knee extension (straightening).

The hamstrings, located on the back of the thigh, are responsible for knee flexion (bending).

The calf muscles (gastrocnemius and soleus) also influence knee flexion and extension.

Other smaller muscles around the knee help control rotational movements. The knee joint allows four basic motions.

Table 3-1 *Summary of the knee kinematics*

Motion	Normal range of motion (Degrees)	Plane of motion
Flexion	0-140	
Extension	0-140 (0-5 degrees of hyperextension)	
Internal rotation	0-15 (with knee flexed)	
External rotation	0-30 (with knee flexed)	

Chapter 3 - The Knee Joint

Flexion:

Bending the knee, bringing the heel toward the buttocks.

Extension:

Straightening the knee from a flexed position.

Internal Rotation:

Rotating the tibia inward (toward the body midline).

External Rotation:

Rotating the tibia outward (away from the midline of the body).

All of these movements involve coordinated actions of the muscles, tendons, and ligaments to ensure smooth and controlled motion within various anatomical planes.

Therefore, the soft tissues surrounding the knee joint, including menisci, tendons, ligaments, and muscles, are essential for enabling movement and maintaining stability.

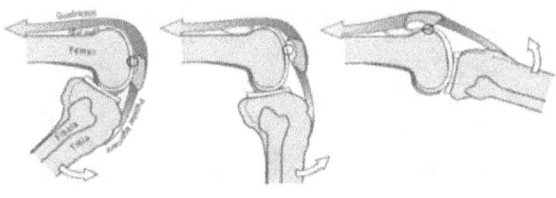

Figure 3-9 *Knee extension motion*

These structures work together to support the four fundamental motions of the knee joint, ensuring that it functions effectively and safely during activities such as walking, running, and other forms of physical activity.

Knee implants

Knee implants are available in a variety of configurations, tailored to address diverse needs and stages in knee replacement surgery.

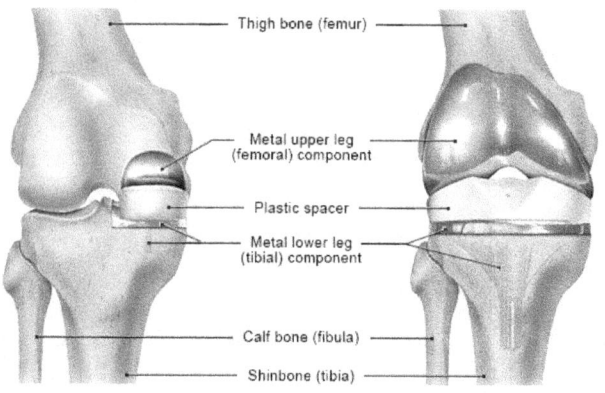

Figure 3-10 *Partial knee vs total knee system*

Beyond revision knee implants, the primary classifications for knee replacement encompass total knee replacement, partial (unicompartmental) knee replacement, bicompartmental knee replacement, and kneecap replacements, which are employed in patellofemoral arthroplasty.

Total Knee Replacement

A total knee replacement (TKR), also known as total knee arthroplasty (TKA), is a surgical procedure aimed at replacing the damaged or arthritic knee joint with artificial components.

These components work together to restore the function and movement of the knee. Here, we'll elaborate on the four main components of a typical TKR, along with occasional additions (augments).

Femoral Component

The femoral component is the uppermost part of the artificial knee joint. It is designed to replace the damaged or worn-out end of the femur (thigh bone).

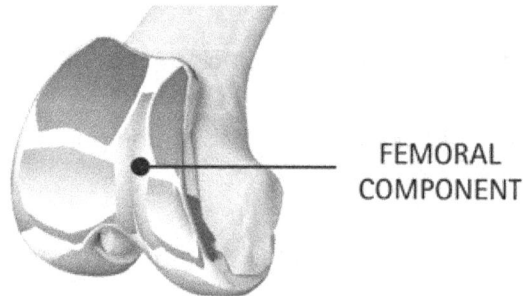

Figure 3-11 *Total knee femoral component*

This component is typically made from durable materials such as metal (often cobalt-chromium alloy) or a combination of metal and ceramic.

Polyethylene Insert

Located in the middle of the TKR, the polyethylene insert serves as the bearing surface between the femoral and tibial components.

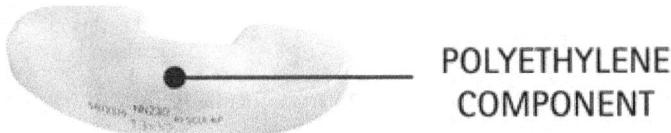

POLYETHYLENE COMPONENT

Figure 3-12 *Total knee polyethylene component or tibial insert or plastic spacer*

It acts as a cushion and provides a smooth articulating surface for the knee joint to move. This insert is made from high-density PE (polyethylene), a tough and wear-resistant plastic.

Tibial Component, Tray or Baseplate

The tibial component, also known as the tibial tray, is the bottom part of the artificial knee joint. It replaces the damaged top surface of the tibia (shin bone).

Like the femoral component, the tibial component is typically constructed from metal or a combination of metal and plastic.

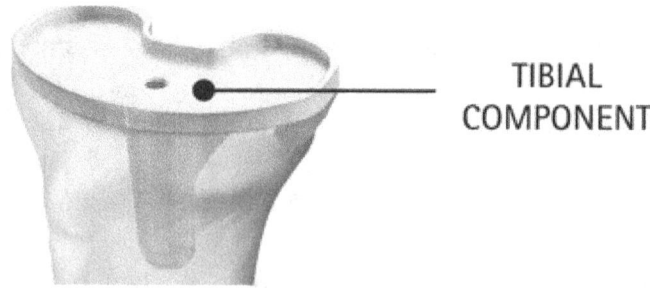

Figure 3-13 *Total knee tibial tray*

Patellar Component

The fourth part of a TKR is the patella or knee cap component.

This component is designed to replace the damaged surface of the kneecap (patella). It provides a smooth articulating surface for the femoral component to interact with when the knee is bent and straightened.

The patellar component can also be made from metal or plastic, depending on the surgeon's choice and the patient's needs.

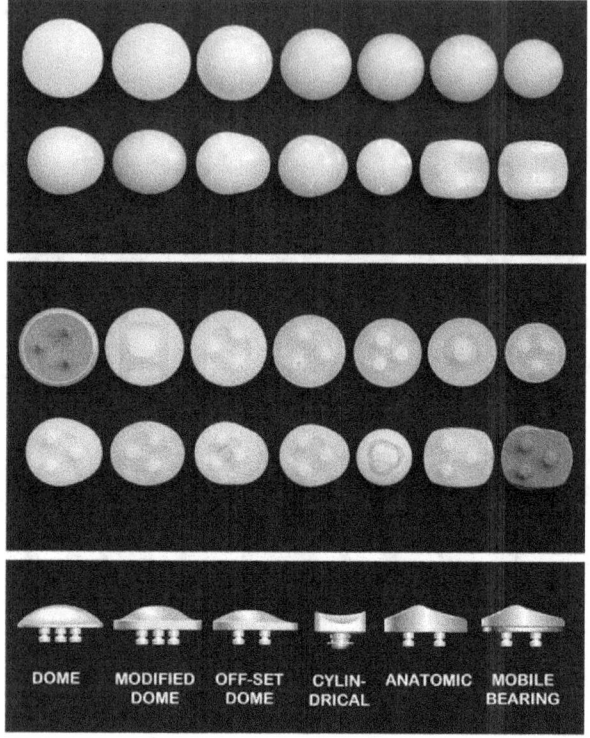

Figure 3-14 *Some examples of TKA patellar component (by Oliver S. Schindler)*

In addition to these four main components, there are occasional additions, such as augments or sleeves, which may be used in specific cases, particularly in revision TKR.

Augments are additional pieces that may be added to the femoral or tibial components to address bone loss or deformities.

For example, a sleeve can be added to enhance the stability of the femoral or tibial component in cases of extensive bone loss.

The primary goal of a total knee replacement is to relieve pain, improve knee joint function, and enhance the patient's overall quality of life.

The choice of components and any additional elements are carefully selected based on the patient's individual condition and the surgeon's assessment to ensure the best possible outcome in terms of knee function and durability.

Partial (Unicompartmental) Knee Replacement

A unicompartmental knee replacement/arthroplasty (UKA), often referred to as a partial knee replacement or uni-knee replacement, is a surgical procedure that involves replacing only one part (compartment) of the knee joint with an artificial implant, rather than replacing the entire knee joint as in a total knee replacement.

This procedure is typically chosen when the damage or arthritis is confined to a specific area of the knee, leaving the other compartments relatively healthy.

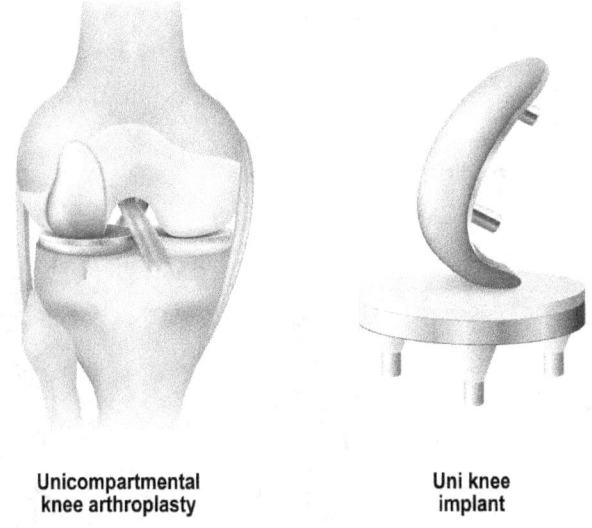

Unicompartmental knee arthroplasty

Uni knee implant

Figure 3-15 *Unicompartmental knee implant*

Uni-knee replacement is most suitable for patients whose knee arthritis or damage is limited to one compartment of the knee joint, either the medial (inner), lateral (outer), or patellofemoral (kneecap) compartment.

Patient selection is critical, and the surgeon carefully evaluates factors such as the extent of joint damage, the location of arthritis, and the patient's overall health to determine if they are a suitable candidate.

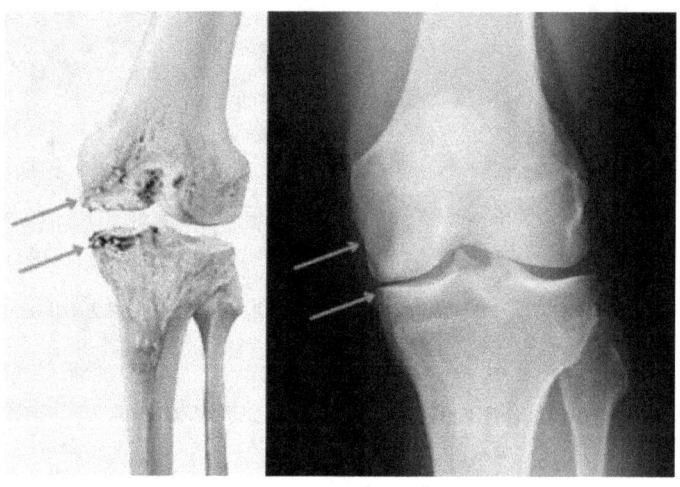

Figure 3-16 *Illustration and X-ray image of medial compartment osteoarthritis of the knee (by Michael M. Alexiades, MD)*

During the surgery, the orthopaedic surgeon removes the damaged portion of the knee joint and replaces it with an artificial implant. This implant typically includes a femoral component which replaces the end of the femur (thigh bone) that articulates with the damaged compartment of the knee.

A polyethylene insert which is placed between the femoral component and the tibial component to provide a smooth and durable bearing surface.

Lastly, there is a tibial component which replaces the top surface of the tibia (shin bone) in the compartment being treated.

Uni-knee replacement offers several advantages over a total knee replacement. For example, there are smaller incisions (compared with TKA), which may result in less post-operative pain and quicker recovery.

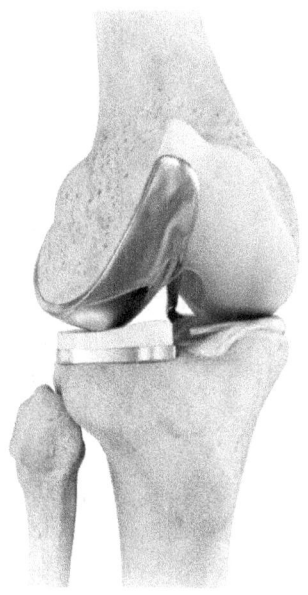

Figure 3-17 *Preservation of healthy knee joint structures, including ligaments and bone, in the non-affected compartments*

Also preservation of healthy knee joint structures, including ligaments and bone, in the non-affected compartments.

There is a potential for a more natural feeling knee with a greater range of motion. And last but not least, reduced blood loss during surgery and shorter hospital stays.

Rehabilitation after a unicompartmental knee replacement is generally faster compared to a total knee replacement.

Physical therapy is an essential part of the recovery process to improve strength, flexibility, and mobility.

Patients can often return to normal daily activities, including low-impact sports, within a shorter timeframe than with a total knee replacement.

It's important to note that not all patients are candidates for unicompartmental or partial knee replacement, and the decision should be made in consultation with an orthopaedic surgeon who specialises in knee joint procedures.

This procedure is most effective when applied to carefully selected patients with isolated compartmental knee damage, offering them the potential for pain relief & improved knee function.

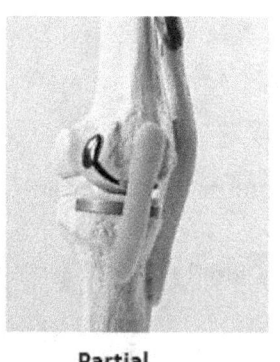
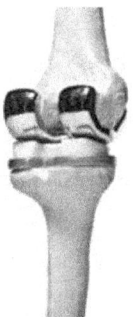

Partial Knee **Total Knee**

Figure 3-18 *UKA & TKA posterior view*

Bicompartmental Knee Replacement

Bicompartmental knee replacement/arthroplasty (BKA) is a surgical approach that replaces two compartments of the knee joint, typically the medial and patellofemoral compartments, while preserving the lateral compartment. It is considered for patients with specific patterns of knee joint wear, such as damage to both the medial and patellofemoral compartments.

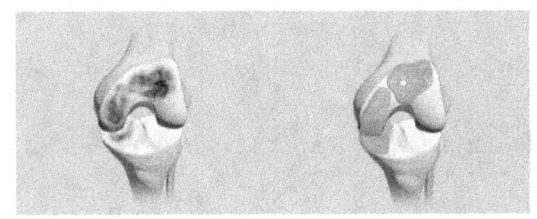

Figure 3-19 *Bicompartmental knee replacement*

Kneecap or Patellofemoral Arthroplasty

Patellofemoral arthroplasty focuses on the replacement of the patellofemoral joint (PFJ), which is the joint between the kneecap (patella) and the front of the thigh bone (femur).

It is designed to address issues specifically in this part of the knee. This procedure is suitable for individuals with isolated patellofemoral joint arthritis or damage.

Each type of knee replacement has its own indications, advantages, and considerations.

The choice of implant and surgical approach is typically determined by the extent and location of knee joint damage, the patient's individual circumstances, and the recommendations of the orthopaedic surgeon.

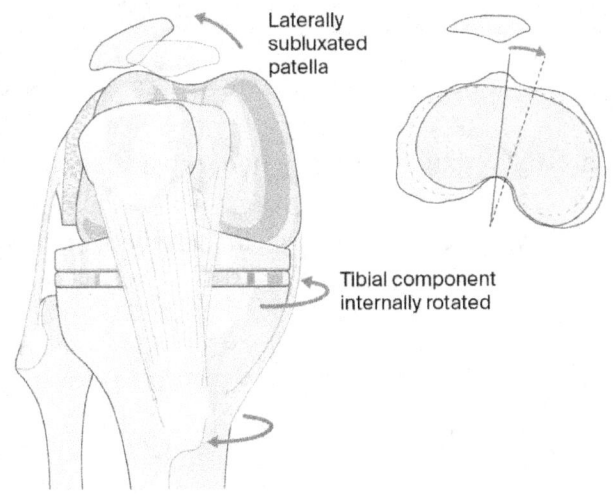

Figure 3-20 *Patellofemoral alignment*

Before moving on to the next section, let's have a quick look at "knee resurfacing". Episealer knee resurfacing is a targeted approach to treat localised cartilage damage in the knee joint, preserving healthy bone and suiting younger, active patients.

Unlike total (or partial) knee replacement, knee resurfacing minimises bone removal, offers shorter recovery times, and is ideal for specific knee areas, while total and uni knee replacements are used for widespread damage in older patients.

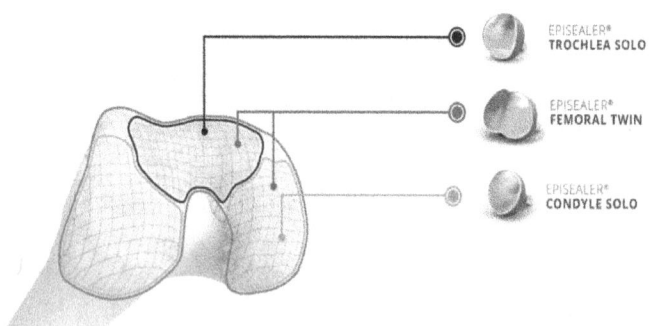

Figure 3-21 *The Episealer Implant*

TKA Implant design and materials

Total knee arthroplasty (TKA) implants come in various designs and materials to cater to the diverse needs of patients.

These options allow orthopaedic surgeons to tailor the implant choice to each individual's unique anatomy and lifestyle.

Design variations may include different types of knee components, such as fixed-bearing or mobile-bearing implants, as well as options for patellar resurfacing.

In terms of materials, TKA implants can be made from metals like cobalt-chromium alloys, ceramics, and highly cross-linked polyethylene.

Each material has its own set of advantages and considerations, allowing surgeons to select the most appropriate implant to optimise longevity, stability, and overall patient satisfaction in knee replacement surgeries.

<u>Femoral Component</u>

The femoral component of a total knee system comprises two surfaces: the fixation surface and the bearing surface. The fixation surface is where the implant attaches to the distal end of the femur.

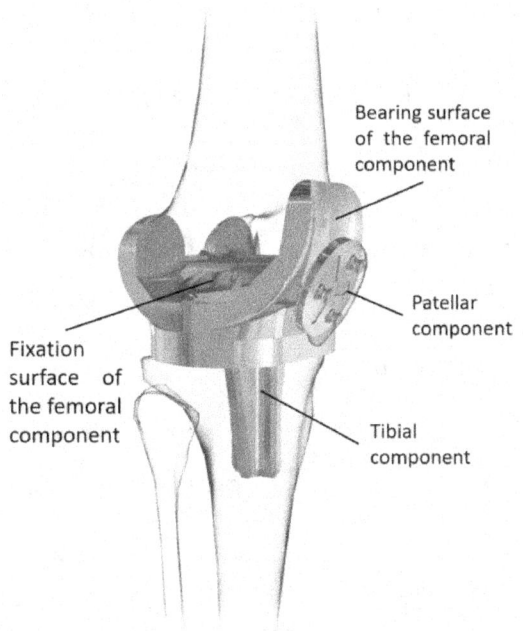

Figure 3-22 *Total knee replacement components*

This attachment can be achieved with bone cement, or in the case of a cementless femoral component, the roughened porous or hydroxyapatite (HA)-coated surface of the fixation area promotes bone ingrowth for secure attachment to the bone.

Conversely, the smooth and polished bearing surface of the femoral component is where articulation into the polyethylene insert occurs, facilitating motion within the knee implant.

Tibial Component

The tibial insert in a total knee replacement system interacts with the tibial component at its base, creating the tibial bearing surface, and aligns with the femoral bearing surface on its upper side.

Two types of tibial components exist: mono-block, where the insert is pre-assembled onto the tibial baseplate, and modular, composed of two separate parts joined by the surgeon during the procedure.

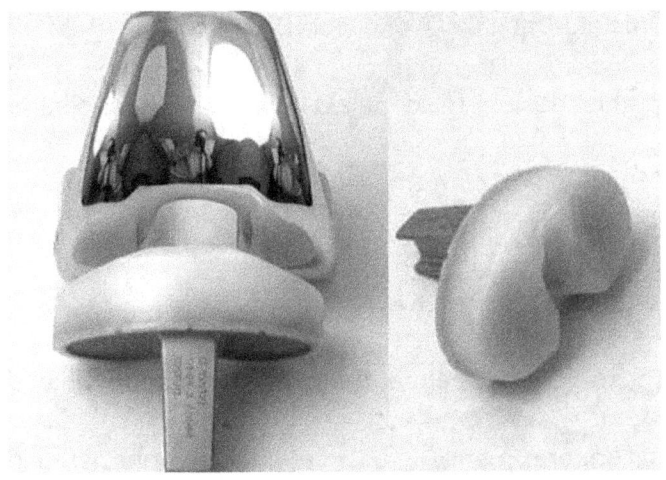

Figure 3-23 *Left: Anatomic Graduated Component (AGC), right: mono block tibial component*

Modular tibial components offer a range of tibial tray and polyethylene (PE) insert designs, which vary according to the configurations of the tibial and femoral bearing surfaces.

Cruciate-Retaining Design:

This design allows for the retention of the posterior cruciate ligament (PCL).

Cruciate-Sacrificing or Deep-Dish Design:

In this design (also called Condylar Stabilising or CS), the PCL is removed.

Anterior Stabilised Design:

These inserts feature a highly conforming anterior lip (approximately 10 mm) to prevent anterior dislocation of the femoral component.

Posterior Stabilised Design:

This design includes a central post and is one of the most commonly used types in TKA implants.

Medially Conforming Ball-and-Socket Design:

This design replicates a healthy knee joint's femoral rollback profile.

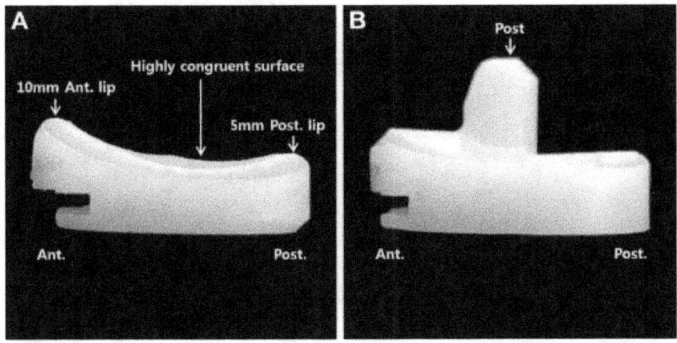

Figure 3-24 A*nterior stabilised (A), and posterior stabilised (B) tibial insert (by Yong In, MD)*

Tibial Insert Design

As mentioned previously, polyethylene (PE) insert design in total knee arthroplasty can be categorised into several main designs listed here.

Surgeon preference for either design depends on the specific wear and range of motion characteristics that are most suitable for each patient.

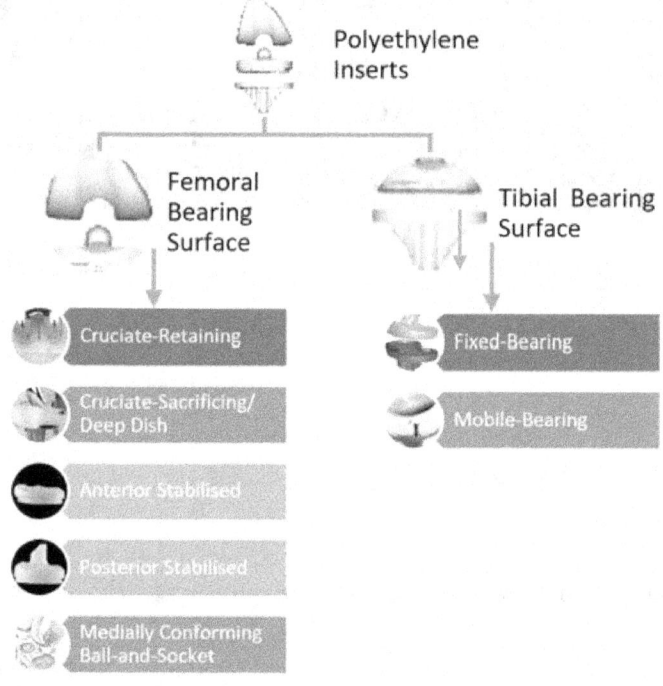

Figure 3-25 *Polyethylene insert types by design*

Posterior-Stabilised (PS) Total Knee System:

This type of TKR system features a post mechanism that replaces the posterior cruciate ligament (PCL).

It provides stability by controlling the rollback of the femur on the tibia during knee flexion. PS systems are commonly used and offer good stability and function for many patients.

Cruciate-Retaining (CR) Total Knee System:
CR TKR systems preserve the PCL, and the implant design is intended to work in harmony with the patient's existing PCL.

These systems are suitable for patients with a well-functioning PCL and are designed to maintain more natural knee kinematics.

Chapter 3 - The Knee Joint

Medial Pivot Total Knee System:

This system is designed to replicate the natural movement of the knee more closely by focusing on the medial compartment.

It aims to provide stability during activities like walking and ascending/descending stairs.

Rotating Platform Total Knee System:

In a rotating platform TKR, the polyethylene insert between the femoral and tibial components can rotate slightly.

This design is intended to mimic the natural rotational movement of the knee and reduce wear on the implant components.

Customised or Patient-Specific Total Knee Systems:

These systems involve the use of patient-specific data, often obtained from pre-operative imaging, to create a customised implant and surgical plan tailored to the individual patient.

This approach can improve the fit and alignment of the implant.

Gender-Specific Total Knee Systems:

Some TKR systems are designed with consideration for gender-specific anatomical differences.

These implants aim to better accommodate the typical size and shape variations between male and female knees.

Highly Cross-Linked Polyethylene (XLPE) Bearing: While not an entire TKR system, the choice of bearing material can greatly impact the longevity of the implant.

Highly cross-linked polyethylene is a type of plastic used for the bearing surfaces, known for its durability and reduced wear rates.

As mentioned before, the selection of a specific TKR system depends on various factors, including the patient's anatomy, age, activity level, and the surgeon's expertise and preferences.

Surgeons carefully evaluate these factors to choose the most appropriate implant and surgical approach for each individual to optimise the outcome of the knee replacement procedure.

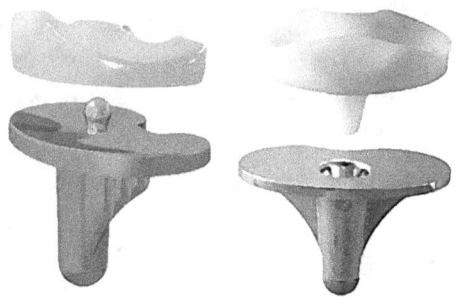

Figure 3-26 *Two mobile bearing designs*

A recent study conducted by Professor Poirier at the University of Western Brittany in France has found that there are no significant differences in clinical outcomes between fixed-bearing & mobile-bearing inserts of the same total knee arthroplasty (TKA) construct.

The Inferior Surface of the Insert (Tibial Locking)

The surface of polyethylene (PE) insert that is fixed onto the metallic tibial baseplate in total knee arthroplasty can be categorised into two main designs: fixed-bearing (FB) and mobile-bearing (MB) systems.

Surgeon preference for either design depends on the specific wear and range of motion characteristics that are most suitable for each patient.

Here you can see the designs for both fixed-bearing (FB) and mobile-bearing (MB) total knee arthroplasty systems. In the FB system, take note of the elevated edge on the tibial component, which is designed to secure the PE insert in place.

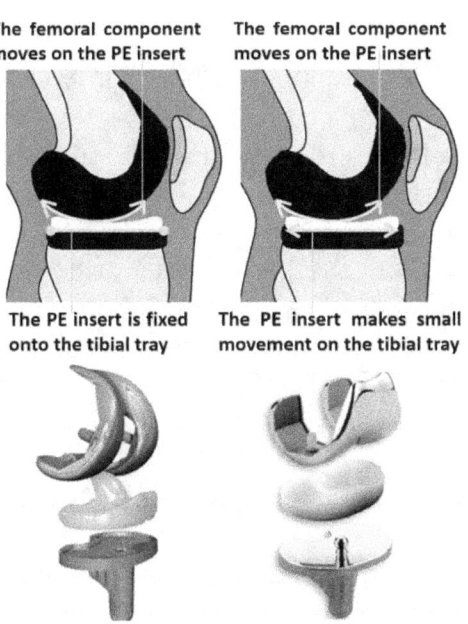

Figure 3-27 *Left: fixed-bearing TKR, right: mobile-bearing or rotating platform (RP) TKR*

The only movement in the FB system occurs between the femoral component and the PE insert. If the insert shifts even slightly against the tibial base, it usually indicates PE fracture or wear, and this would necessitate a revision surgery for the knee.

On the other hand, in the mobile-bearing or rotating platform (RP) design, the primary motion for flexion and extension occurs between the femoral component and the PE insert.

However, in this system, the PE insert is not fixed onto the tibial tray, allowing it to rotate against the smooth surface of the tibial component. This design introduces a risk of the connection mechanism's stem fracturing.

Modular Tibial Tray or Baseplate

The tibial tray or tibial component is designed to be affixed to the proximal tibia using a short stem that fits into the tibial medullary canal, providing a surface for the PE insert to rest on.

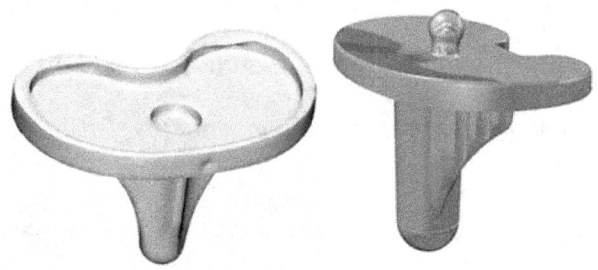

Figure 3-28 *Two TKR tibial tray designs, fixed bearing & rotating platform*

The tibial component has two surfaces: a bearing surface that interacts with the PE insert and a

211

fixation surface, which can be implanted using either a cemented or a cementless approach.

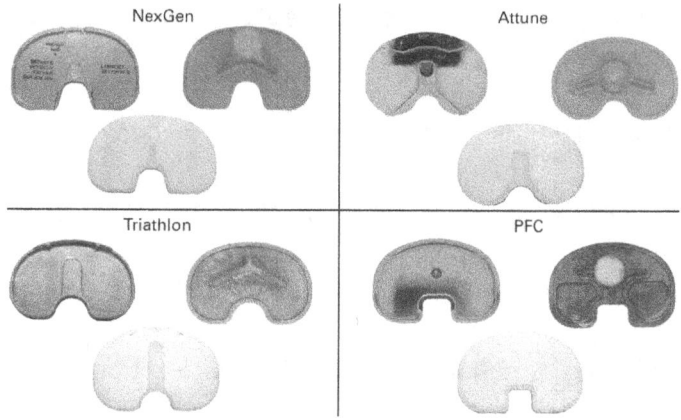

Figure 3-29 *Top & bottom view of 4 separate tibial components (Nexgen, Attune, Triathlon, PFC) & their corresponding PE inserts (by R.Bhalekar)*

Lastly, and as previously highlighted the patellar component is an all-polyethylene or metal and PE dome with a fixation surface that is attached to the patellar bone, either with or without the use of bone cement.

Primary vs. Revision Knee Implants

Revision surgery for knee implants is necessary when the original knee implant, whether it's a TKR or UKR, is no longer functioning properly.

This can occur due to a variety of reasons, including implant wear, loosening, infection, instability, implant breakage, or other complications.

The goal of revision surgery is to replace the existing implant to restore function, reduce pain, and improve the patient's quality of life.

In primary total knee replacements, a patient typically undergoes the procedure for one knee (unilateral TKR) or both knees (bilateral TKR) simultaneously or in separate surgeries.

However, revision surgeries differ in that they are performed after the initial knee replacement.

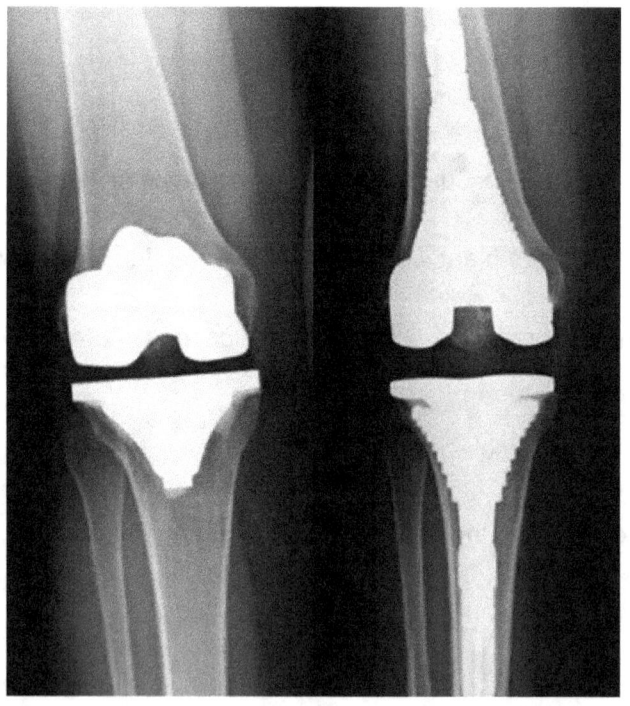

Figure 3-30 *Left: primary total knee replacement, right: revision TKR*

Any subsequent surgeries on the same knee(s), whether it's the same knee or the other knee, are considered revision knee replacements. This means that a patient can potentially undergo multiple revision surgeries if necessary.

Revision surgery is generally considered more complex and challenging than primary knee replacement for several reasons:

- Bone Loss - Managing bone loss is a critical aspect of revision knee replacements. The bone around the knee joint may have already been compromised due to the initial surgery, implant wear, or other factors. Additionally, the revision surgery itself can lead to further bone loss as the surgeon removes and replaces the original implant components.

- Complex Anatomy - Revision surgeries often involve dealing with altered anatomy, which can make the procedure more intricate. This may include adjusting the alignment of the components, addressing soft tissue deficiencies, or using specialised implants designed for revision cases.

- Infection Risk - Revision surgeries carry a higher risk of infection compared to primary surgeries, as the presence of the previous implant and associated scar tissue can create a more challenging environment for infection control.

- Implant Selection - The choice of revision implant components is crucial, and surgeons may use larger or more specialised components to address the specific needs of the patient and any bone loss.

It's important to note that bone loss can be either present before the revision surgery (pre-existing) or created during the revision operation itself (induced).

Pre-existing bone loss may result from the complications that led to the revision, while induced bone loss can occur during the process of removing the old implant and preparing the bone for the new components. Managing bone loss often involves using bone grafts or specialised implants to restore stability and function.

Therefore, revision surgery for knee implants is a complex and challenging procedure performed to replace a malfunctioning or deteriorating knee implant.

It distinguishes itself from primary knee replacement in that it occurs after the initial surgery and may involve multiple revisions.

Last but not lease, managing bone loss is a critical aspect of these surgeries, whether it's present before the revision or created during the procedure and requires specialised techniques and implants to achieve a successful outcome.

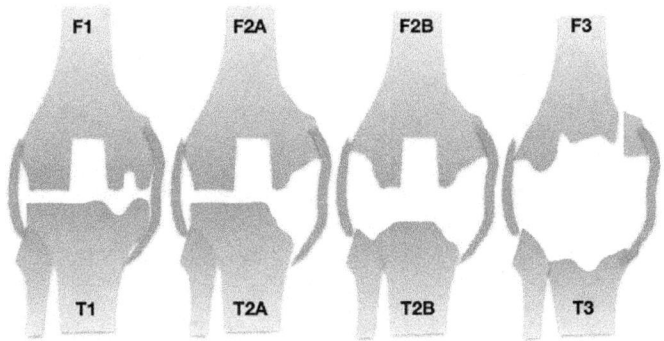

Figure 3-31 *Four degrees* of bone loss in revision total knee arthroplasty

Methods for managing bone loss have traditionally been cement augmentation, impaction bone grafting, bulk structural bone graft and stemmed implants with metal augments. No single technique was found to be superior.

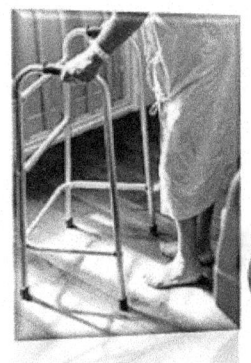
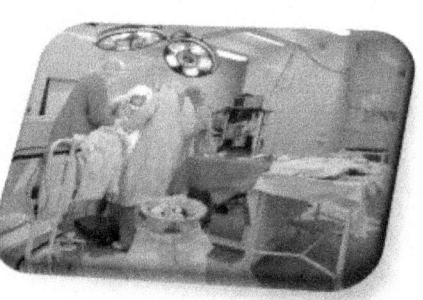

Chapter 4
Joint Replacement Journey

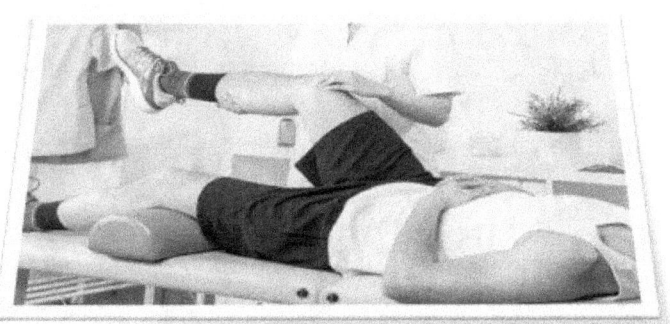

Pre-operative Preparation

Preparing for a joint replacement operation is an important step in ensuring a successful outcome.

In this chapter, you will find a few lists containing some key points to consider before your joint replacement surgery.

Remember, research and education is key. Give yourself plenty time to research and learn general information about the procedure.

Understanding what to expect during and after surgery can help alleviate anxiety and set realistic expectations. Ask your doctor any questions you may have.

Another important factor is consultation. Discuss the surgery thoroughly with your doctor. Understand the reasons for the surgery, the expected benefits, and any potential risks or complications.

It is important to have a clear understanding of the procedure itself.

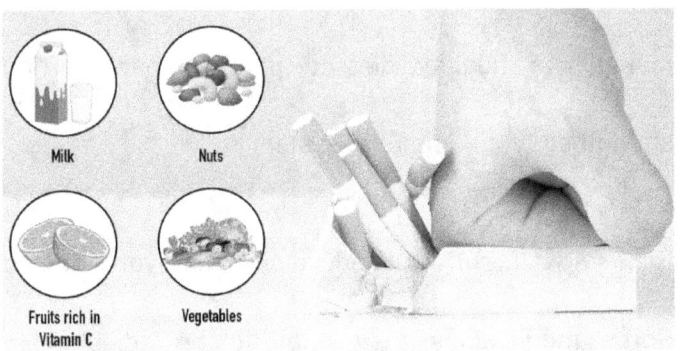

Figure 4-1 *Better your lifestyle (by Dr. Sangeeta)*

Physical Preparation

Follow your doctor's recommendations for any preoperative exercises or physical therapy to help strengthen the muscles around your joint and improve your overall physical condition.

If you smoke, consider quitting or reducing your smoking as it can impact your healing process.

Maintain a healthy diet to promote healing and strengthen your immune system.

Review your current medications with your doctor. Some medications may need to be adjusted or temporarily stopped before surgery.

Home Preparation

Make necessary modifications to your home to accommodate your needs post-surgery. This may include installing handrails, adjusting the height of chairs and toilets, and removing tripping hazards. Prepare a comfortable recovery area with easy access to necessary items.

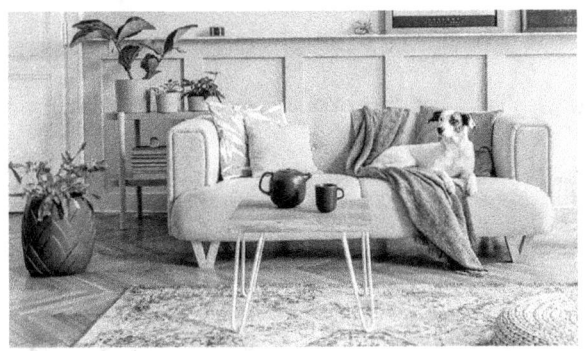

Figure 4-2 *A cluttered living area makes it hard to move with a walking frame*

Chapter 4 - Joint Replacement Journey

Other preparations

Support Network - Tell all your family and close friends about your upcoming surgery. Arrange for someone to assist you after the surgery, especially during the initial days of recovery.

This could be a family member, friend, or hired caregiver.

Preoperative Tests - Your doctor may require you to undergo some preoperative tests, such as blood tests and imaging scans, to assess your overall health and the condition of your joint.

Pre-op Fasting - Follow your doctor's instructions regarding fasting before the surgery. Typically, you will need to avoid eating or drinking for a specified period before the operation.

Clothing - Wear comfortable and loose-fitting clothing on the day of surgery.

Mental Preparation - Prepare yourself mentally for the surgery and the recovery process. Staying positive and focused on the benefits of the surgery can help reduce anxiety.

Dental Clearance - It's best not to have any dental work done within four weeks before hip or knee replacement surgery. Dental issues, like infections, too close to the planned surgery date might lead to a delay in the operation.

One significant risk after surgery is bacterial infection. Bacteria can get into the joint during or after the procedure, and there's also a risk of existing bacteria in the body reaching the site of the artificial joint through the bloodstream.

Doctors and dentists collaborate to reduce the risk of infection.

Pre-op Nail Treatment - Prior to the day of the surgery, it's crucial to be cautious in nail salons, as they may not be the most hygienic of environments and there is usually a risk of skin injury followed by infection during manicure/pedicure treatments.

Avoid acrylic or gel nails, as even a simple nail polish can interfere with monitoring devices like the pulse oximeter during surgery, preventing accurate readings.

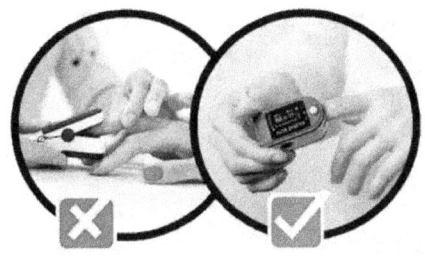

Figure 4-3 *No paint on nails during surgery*

Legal and Financial Matters - Review any legal or financial matters that need attention before your surgery, such as insurance coverage and medical directives.

Chapter 4 - Joint Replacement Journey

Preparing Your Post-op Living Environment

Preparing your home and surroundings for your joint replacement surgery is crucial to ensure a safe and comfortable recovery.

Especially due to having to use a walking frame or a walking stick during the first few days after the surgery.

You'd need to make sure there's enough room for moving in most rooms in your house.

Next is a list of additional considerations and tips for preparing your living environment, in advance of your upcoming joint replacement surgery.

Home Safety Checklist

Declutter - Remove any items or clutter that could obstruct your movement. Ensure clear pathways both inside and outside your home. For example, remove any decorative plant pots off your stairs.

Secure Carpets and Rugs - Fasten or remove loose carpets and rugs to prevent tripping.

Cables and Wires - Tuck away or secure cables and wires to minimise the risk of tripping or falling down.

Chapter 4 - Joint Replacement Journey

Proper Lighting - Install additional lighting in areas you'll be using during the night. Sensor lights can be a convenient addition.

Stairs - Install handrails on both sides of stairs, both indoors and outdoors. Ensure that they are securely fastened.

Bathroom Safety - Make necessary modifications in the bathroom. A few suggestions:

- Install grab bars & handrails in the shower/bath.
- Replace your bathmat with a non-slip mat.
- Get a raised toilet seat to ease sitting/standing.
- Ensure toilet paper is easily accessible.

Accessibility - Place commonly used items within easy reach. Rearrange kitchen items, so you don't need to stretch or bend to access them.

Follow Preoperative Instructions - Adhere to any preoperative instructions provided by your surgeon, including fasting guidelines.

In summary, declutter pathways, secure carpets, install lighting, enhance bathroom safety, and optimise accessibility for daily items.

By taking the above steps to prepare your environment, you can reduce the risk of accidents or discomfort during your recovery. This will also help you create a safer and more supportive space for yourself in your healing journey.

The Patient on the Day of the Surgery

Firstly, remember that each patient's situation is unique, and your doctor will provide you with personalised guidance based on your specific needs and circumstances.

Open communication with your healthcare team is essential throughout the process (starting before the day of your surgery).

Also, the night before your surgery, you may wish to use a marker (thick black head), to draw an arrow on your leg pointing to the joint that is damaged (required a replacement).

Some patients find this method reassuring or calming.

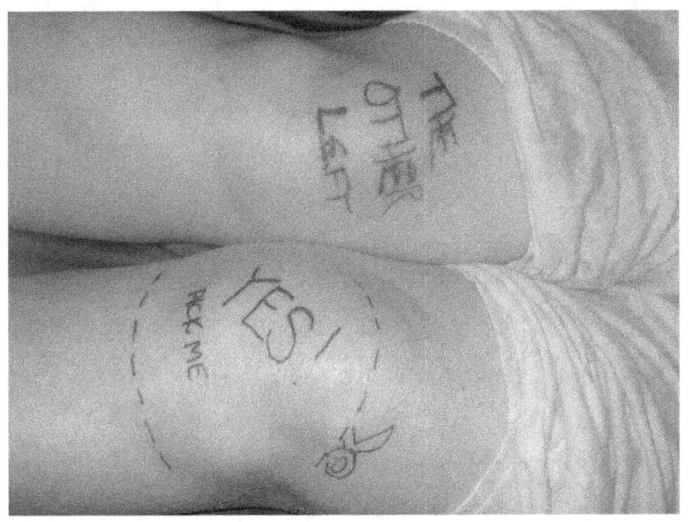

Figure 4-4 *Mark the correct joint*

Preparing for your joint replacement surgery involves careful planning, especially on the day of the operation.

Here are some key considerations and items to remember:

Chapter 4 - Joint Replacement Journey

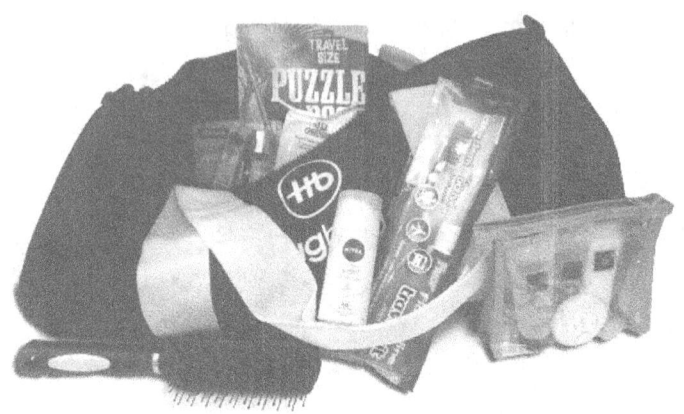

Figure 4-5 *Overnight Hospital Bag by Hugbag*

Overnight Hospital Bag - Check with your surgeon whether you are likely to stay overnight in the hospital.

If so, consider packing an overnight bag with essentials. These may include:

• Toothbrush and toothpaste

• Deodorant

• Dry shampoo (for haircare without water)

- Slip-on shoes (easier to put on)

- Loose-fitting underwear (possible swelling)

- Comfortable clothing (oversized pyjama sets)

- Charger for your mobile phone or tablet

- Headphones or earplugs to help with noise (noisy snoring neighbours) in the hospital

- Menstrual pads instead of a cup or tampons

Makeup and Nails - On the day of the surgery, makeup and nail polish hinder the ability to monitor oxygen levels and can impact the effectiveness of medical tape.

Additionally, many perfumes contain alcohol, posing a risk during surgery where electrical equipment is used, as alcohol-based perfumes can contribute to the spread of fire and cause

Chapter 4 - Joint Replacement Journey

extensive burns. Also, you would need to remove any hair extensions.

Preoperative Holding Area - Your journey on the day of surgery begins in the preoperative holding area, where patients wait before their procedures. An operating room nurse will accompany you to the operating theatre.

Confirmation of Details - Throughout the day, you will be asked to confirm your personal information, including your name, date of birth, type of surgery, and your surgeon's name.

These checks are standard safety procedures. Please stay calm and answer their questions patiently.

Meeting the Surgical Team - When you arrive in the operating theatre, you will see several members of your surgical team preparing for the procedure. This team typically includes:

- Surgical technician
- Anaesthesiologist
- Nurse anaesthetist
- Operating room nurse
- Surgeon
- Physician assistant
- Possibly a medical device representative

Positioning and Preparation - The surgical team will position and prepare you for surgery. They will ensure your comfort and safety throughout the process.

Chapter 4 - Joint Replacement Journey

Surgery and Updates - Your surgery will proceed, and during this time, your family or friends in the waiting area may receive updates from the surgical team.

Your family and friends may be informed when the surgery begins and when you are in the recovery room.

Remember to stay patient and cooperative throughout these procedures, as they are crucial for your safety.

Your surgical team will take all necessary precautions to ensure a successful surgery and a smooth recovery.

Medical Team On the Day of the Surgery

Behind the scenes of your joint replacement surgery, your surgical team conducts extensive preparations to ensure your safety and the success of the procedure.

Here's a glimpse of what happens before you arrive in the operating theatre. Multiple safety checks are performed, and discussions take place before the surgery begins. These checks include:

- Reviewing your personal information, such as your full name, date of birth, and patient reference or identification number.

- Confirming the type of replacement procedure (e.g., hip or knee) and whether it's on the left or right leg.

- Carefully examining your X-rays to ensure a clear understanding of your joint's condition.

- Discussing the medications you are scheduled to receive before the operation, such as antibiotics.

- Reviewing your medical records for any documented allergies.

Allergies are also a crucial consideration. For example, if a patient is allergic to latex, the surgical team takes special precautions.

They will verify and confirm that everyone in the surgical team is wearing latex-free surgical gloves before the operation begins.

Checking the hospital or clinic's inventory or storage room for orthopaedic implants and making sure the implants, trials and instruments required for the surgery are all available.

These meticulous checks and preparations are vital to ensure your safety, prevent complications, and facilitate a smooth surgical process.

They are an essential part of the behind-the-scenes work that goes into your joint replacement surgery.

Chapter 4 - Joint Replacement Journey

Post-op Journey

Recovery from joint replacement surgery is indeed a marathon, and it's important to approach it with patience, a positive attitude, and realistic expectations.

Here are some key points to keep in mind after your joint replacement operation:

Firstly, stay positive! Understand that joint replacement is a major surgery, and it takes time to heal. Maintain a positive attitude throughout your recovery process, and be patient with your body.

Avoid comparing your recovery progress to others who have undergone similar surgeries.

Everyone's medical history and surgical experiences are unique, so your recovery timeline is expected to be different from others.

Communicate with and trust your surgeon! While online resources can be informative, always consult with your surgeon for accurate information and advice tailored to your specific situation.

Your surgeon knows your medical history and can provide guidance accordingly.

Remember, your surgeon is also putting their time and effort to make your joint replacement a

Chapter 4 - Joint Replacement Journey

successful experience for both the patient (you) and his or her own reputation.

Give it some good thought and aim for some realistic expectations. Don't set overly ambitious goals for yourself, such as walking unaided immediately after surgery.

Recovery times vary, and it's important to listen to your body and follow your surgeon's recommendations.

Early mobilisation is key. You may be encouraged to start walking with a walker shortly after surgery.

Early mobilisation is essential for a quicker recovery and to use your new joint effectively.

Rest and activity balance! Find a balance between staying active and allowing your body to rest. Post-surgery fatigue is normal, so listen to your body, rest or nap when needed.

Understand that your recovery and pain reduction take time and long-term commitment to your overall health.

Returning to preoperative activities won't happen immediately.

Besides scheduled physical therapy sessions, home exercises are crucial for strengthening muscles and reducing joint pain.

Follow your prescribed exercises diligently.

As previously mentioned, during the initial months post-surgery, it is advisable to stay mostly at home.

This makes it impractical to go out to a beauty salon for any nail or beauty treatments. Besides that, there are two other challenges when getting the nails done post-operation.

First, getting onto a chair can be challenging, and second, extended hip or knee bending can be painful.

When you do decide to go out, caution the technician to be extra careful to prevent any skin breaks.

It is important to note that nail salons may not be the most sanitary places, and caution is needed to avoid potential infections both before and after the operation.

On a separate note, the number one unmet need in joint replacement recovery is nutrition.

Usually after a major surgical operation patients tend to lose appetite and lose weight for between 4 to 6 weeks post-op (although losing weight may sound like a positive thing, it definitely isn't a good thing here)!

There are studies suggesting this could be linked to increased risk of post-operative infection.

Chapter 4 - Joint Replacement Journey

So it is highly recommended that all joint replacement patients have a nutritious diet for just the period of 6 weeks after the surgery (one may not want to continue longer and gain weight either), because otherwise they may not meet their body's demands through their regular diet alone.

This would enable the body to heal quicker and have better wounds, less swelling and reduced risk of infection.

By maintaining a good diet, a positive mindset, seeking guidance from your surgeon, and committing to your rehabilitation, you can improve your chances of a successful and satisfying recovery.

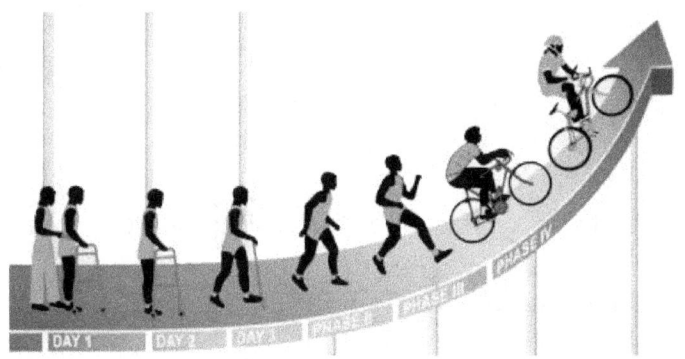

Figure 4-6 *Recovering from joint replacement is like a marathon, not a sprint, requiring time and dedication!*

Remember, after joint replacement surgery, mobility can be limited in the initial days, so making modifications to your walking aid to carry essential items like your mobile phone or water bottle can be very helpful.

A few more tips to consider

- Purchase or Make a Necessities Pouch - You can make a small pouch or bag that can be attached to your walker or crutches. This pouch can hold items like your phone, water bottle, medications, tissues, and other essentials you may need while moving around the house.

- Keep Items at Waist Height - Ensure that any items you frequently need are within easy reach, ideally at waist height. You can use a small table or shelf next to your chair or bed to keep these items accessible. Remember not to leave anything you'd need on the floor.

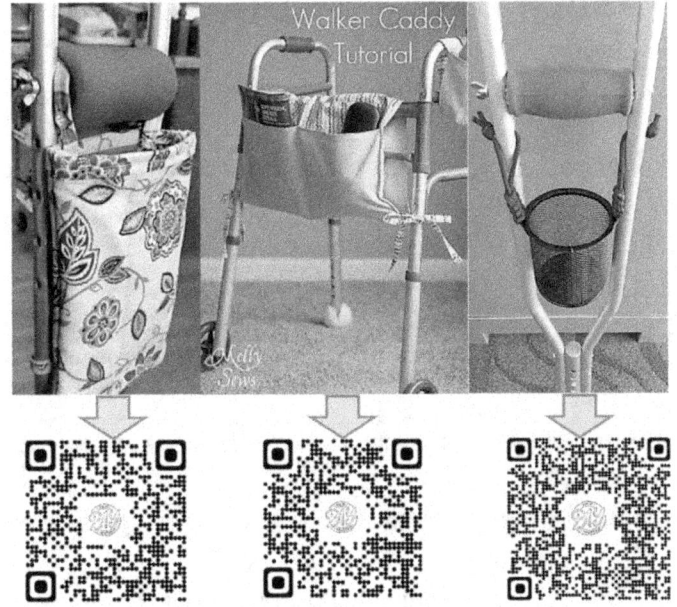

Figure 4-7 *Examples of the DIY little bag, caddy and water bottle holder for walking aids (scan the corresponding QR codes to access each website/tutorial)*

- Ask for Help - If you have friends or family members around, don't hesitate to ask for assistance with tasks that may be challenging during your early recovery days.

Chapter 4 - Joint Replacement Journey

- Use a Backpack - Consider wearing a lightweight backpack when using your walker or crutches. This can provide additional storage for items you need to carry around.

- Maintain a Safe Environment - Ensure that your home is free of tripping hazards, loose rugs, or cluttered areas that can make moving around more difficult. Especially during your early days after the surgery when you'll be using a walking frame. Also, install handrails or safety bars where needed, especially in the bathroom.

- Plan Ahead - Before surgery, plan and organise your living space to make it as convenient as possible for your recovery period. This includes rearranging furniture to create clear pathways and removing obstacles.

- Remember that adapting your living space and mobility aids to your needs can greatly enhance your comfort and independence during the early stages of your recovery.

- Scars and Appearance - It's common to be concerned about the appearance of surgical scars. Keep in mind that scars typically fade over time. You can also use scar creams or silicone sheets, (double-check with your surgeon), to help minimise their appearance. Most importantly, these scars are a testament to your journey toward improved joint health.

- Hair on Legs - Shaving your legs may be challenging during the early stages of recovery. If this is a concern, you might consider using an electric razor or asking for assistance from a family member or caregiver. However, it's essential to prioritise your safety and comfort over cosmetic concerns during this recovery period.

- Pet Safety - Pets are indeed a wonderful source of comfort, but their presence can pose certain risks during your recovery. To prevent accidents, take your time when walking around pets, especially if they are excited and may jump or run near you. Having someone help with pet care during your initial recovery period is an excellent idea.

- Post-Operation Precautions - Following your surgeon's instructions and precautions is crucial for a successful recovery. These guidelines are designed to protect your new joint and ensure its proper healing. It's important not to rush into activities that could strain or damage your joint. Always listen to your body!

- Occupational Therapy - In some cases, occupational therapy can be beneficial after joint replacement surgery. An occupational therapist can provide practical tips and techniques for daily activities, such as dressing, bathing, and cooking, while protecting your new joint.

Chapter 4 - Joint Replacement Journey

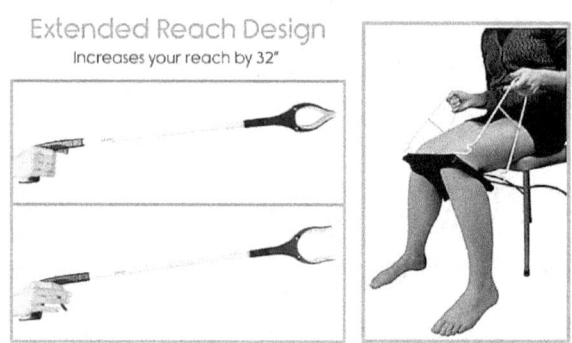

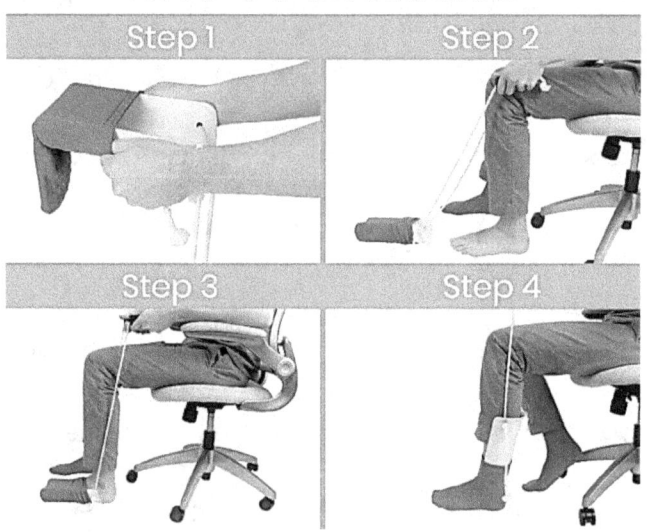

Figure 4-8 *Top left: picking up or reaching assist tool, top right: pants lift and slip aid, bottom: sock aid device. All available to purchase online*

Post-Operative (After Surgery) General Instructions

Here are some valuable tips for those who have undergone hip or knee replacement surgery. Managing daily activities and social engagements after joint replacement can be challenging during the early stages of recovery.

- Seating Arrangements - Planning ahead for seating in various situations is an excellent strategy. When attending events or gatherings, choosing seats near exits or aisles allows for more flexibility and ease of movement. Many venues and theatres offer accessible seating options, which can be particularly beneficial for those with a joint replacement.

- Mobility Aids - Some people find that using a cane or a walking aid for a brief period during social gatherings or events can provide additional support and stability, especially when navigating crowded or unfamiliar places.

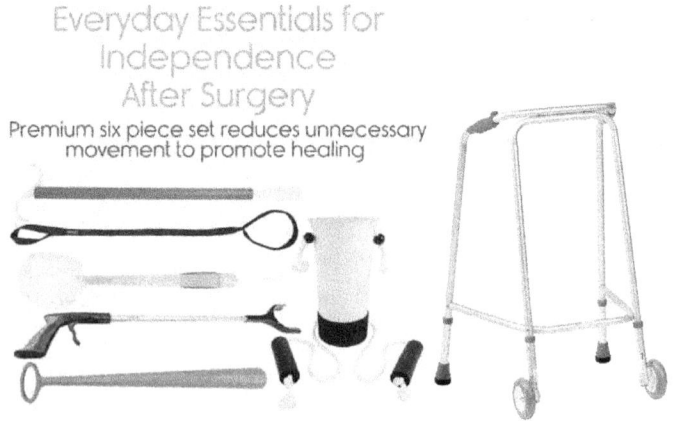

Figure 4-9 *Mobility aids*

- Medication Management - If you experience discomfort or stiffness when sitting for extended periods, consider taking any prescribed pain medications as directed by your healthcare provider before such events. However, always consult your surgeon or healthcare provider regarding medication use.

- Stretching and Movement - Gentle stretches and range-of-motion exercises during breaks can help alleviate discomfort and maintain joint flexibility. Consult your medical team or physical therapist for guidance on specific exercises that can be incorporated into your routine.

- Communication - Don't hesitate to inform event organisers or airline staff about your condition and any special needs you may have. They may be able to provide accommodations or assistance to ensure your comfort and safety.

- Footwear - Choosing comfortable and supportive footwear can make a significant difference in reducing joint discomfort, especially when you need to be on your feet for extended periods.

Ultimately, the goal is to strike a balance between maintaining an active & fulfilling lifestyle while safeguarding the integrity of your newly replaced joint. Listening to your body, staying prepared, and seeking accommodations when necessary can help you enjoy social activities and events while managing any challenges that may arise during the recovery process.

Revision THA/TKA

Joint replacement revision, which involves replacing or repairing a previously implanted joint prosthesis, is a complex procedure that can be influenced by various factors.

Here are some key points to consider regarding revision joint replacement:

Causes for Revision - Joint replacement revisions are typically performed due to various reasons.

Reasons including aseptic loosening (when the implant becomes loose without infection), adverse soft tissue reactions to wear particles, dislocation or subluxation (partial dislocation), persistent pain, and infection. These issues can result from factors such as implant wear and tear, implant design, patient factors, or surgical technique.

Implant Longevity - The longevity of a joint replacement implant depends on multiple factors, including the type of implant used, patient activity level, and implant wear characteristics.

Advances in implant materials and design have extended the lifespan of joint replacements, but they are not permanent solutions and may eventually require revision.

Patient Factors - Patient-related factors such as age, overall health, BMI (Body Mass Index), and medical history can impact the success of a joint replacement and the likelihood of a revision. Maintaining a healthy lifestyle, including weight management and staying active within the recommended limits, can contribute to implant longevity.

Surgical Expertise - The success of a joint replacement revision heavily relies on the skills and experience of the orthopaedic surgeon performing the procedure. Surgeons must carefully assess the patient's condition, address any complications, and select the appropriate revision components.

Infection Control - Infection is a significant concern in joint replacement revisions. Adequate infection control measures are essential during the revision surgery to minimise the risk of post-operative infections.

Rehabilitation and Recovery - The rehabilitation process after joint replacement revision is often more challenging than after the initial joint replacement surgery. Patients may require longer recovery periods and more intensive physical therapy to regain function and mobility.

Patient Education - Educating patients about the importance of follow-up appointments, implant care, and recognising signs of potential complications is crucial in preventing revision surgery.

Registry Data - National joint registries, like the UK's National Joint Registry, provide valuable data on the performance and outcomes of joint replacement surgeries. This data helps identify trends, improve implant designs, and enhance patient care.

Joint replacement revision is a complex and specialised procedure that aims to address issues and improve the function and comfort of individuals who have undergone joint replacement.

Careful monitoring, prompt intervention when complications arise, and a collaborative approach between patients and healthcare providers are essential components of successful joint replacement revision outcomes.

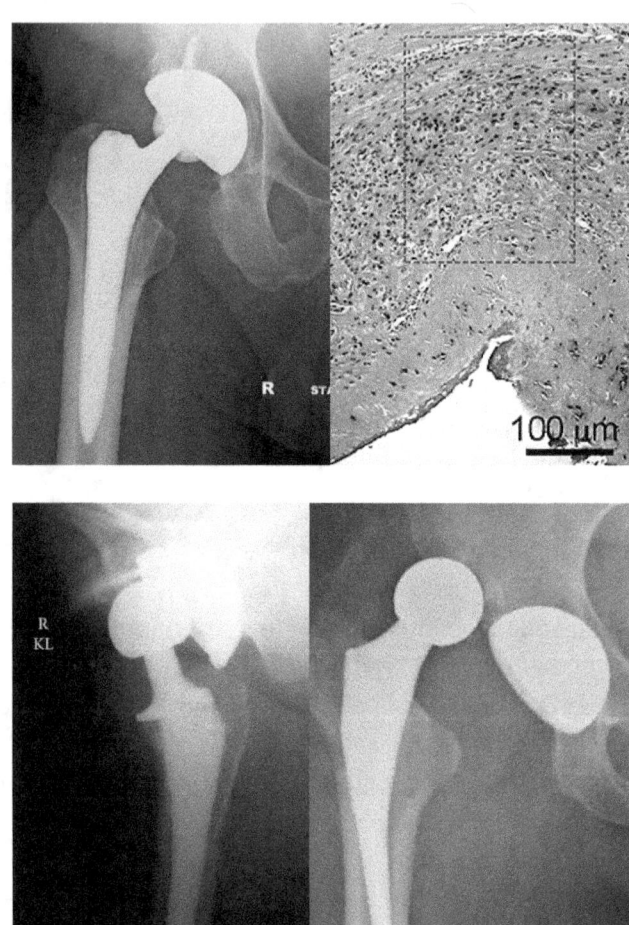

Figure 4-10 *Top left: aseptic loosening of the stem, right: adverse tissue reaction to debris, bottom left: subluxation or partial dislocation, right: dislocation of the right hip head*

Common Reasons for Revision

The data from the UK's National Joint Registry (NJR) highlights some of the most common reasons for revision hip replacements. Here's a brief explanation of each:

- Aseptic Loosening - Aseptic loosening occurs when the components of the hip implant become loose over time without an active infection. This can lead to pain, instability, and reduced function. Revision surgery is needed to address this issue by replacing the loosened components.

- Dislocation or Subluxation - Dislocation involves the complete separation of the hip joint's components, while subluxation refers to a partial dislocation. These often result from instability of the implant, & they can cause discomfort and functional limitations. Revision aims to stabilise the joint & reduce the risk of further dislocations.

- Adverse Soft Tissue Reaction - Adverse soft tissue reactions are typically caused by wear particles generated by the implant's components. These particles can trigger an inflammatory response in the surrounding soft tissues, leading to pain and discomfort. Revision surgery may involve changing implant components to reduce wear and inflammation.

- Pain - Persistent or severe pain after a hip replacement is an indication that something may be wrong with the implant or its surrounding tissues. The cause of the pain needs to be carefully diagnosed, and revision surgery may be required to address the underlying issue.

- Infection - Infection can occur at any time following a hip replacement, and it can lead to severe complications. Revision is necessary to remove infected tissues, replace the implant, and administer antibiotics to clear the infection.

- Lysis (Osteolysis) - Osteolysis refers to the loss of bone around the implant due to wear and debris, which can also result in loosening and discomfort. Revision surgery is typically required to address these issues.

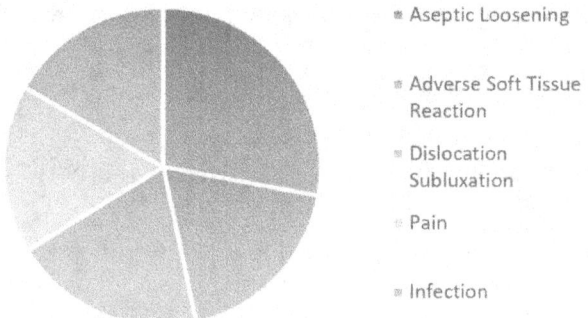

Figure 4-11 *Top reasons for revision THR*

- Progressive Arthritis - Progressive arthritis in the patellofemoral joint can occur over time, even after a primary replacement. This can lead to discomfort, & instability. Revision may involve changing the implant to address arthritis.

- Instability - Joint instability can result from various factors, including issues with implant positioning, soft tissue imbalances, or wear and tear. Revision surgery aims to restore stability and improve joint function.

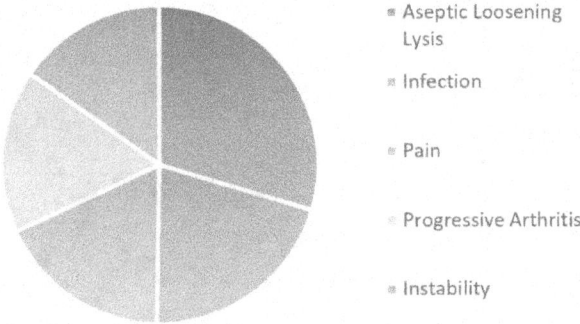

Figure 4-12 *Top reasons for revision TKR*

These common reasons for revision highlight the importance of thorough evaluation, accurate diagnosis, and appropriate surgical intervention when issues arise. Regular follow-up and monitoring are essential to detect and address problems early, ultimately leading to better outcomes for patients.

Chapter 4 - Joint Replacement Journey

Chapter 5
Appendices

Appendix 1 - Glossary

Acrylic: a type of cloth or plastic produced by chemical processes.

Alignment: an arrangement in which two or more things are positioned in a straight line or parallel to each other.

Angle of inclination: the angle between the equatorial plane of the earth and the orbital plane of the satellite.

Ankle [Dorsiflexion vs. Plantarflexion]: two of the main ankle movements as shown below.

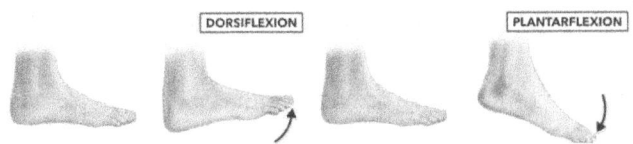

Arthritis: a serious condition in which a person's joints (= the places where two bones are connected) become painful, swollen, and stiff.

Arthroplasty: literally means [re]forming of joint, the surgical reconstruction or replacement of a joint.

Aseptic loosening: is the failure of the bond between an implant and bone in the absence of infection (aseptic).

Augment: to make something larger or fuller by adding something to it.

Biocompatible: (especially of material used in surgical implants) not harmful or toxic to living tissue.

BMI: abbreviation for body mass index: a measurement of someone's weight in relation to their height.

Bone cement: Polymethyl methacrylate (PMMA), is commonly known as bone cement, and is widely used for implant fixation in various Orthopaedic and trauma surgery.

Cemented: Bone cement was used for implant fixation.

Cementless: Bone cement was not used for implant fixation.

Complex joint: a joint composed of three or more skeletal elements, or in which two anatomically separate joints function as a unit.

Congruent: (of figures) identical in form; coinciding exactly when superimposed.

Corrosion: surface degradation due to electrochemical interactions producing metallic ions and salts which applies only to metals.

Debris: particles of different material and size shed from the surface of the various parts of the implant due to wear.

Distal: away from the centre of the body or from the point of attachment to a bone or muscle. Opposite to proximal.

Driver: something that makes other things progress, develop, or grow stronger.

Epidemic: the appearance of a particular disease in a large number of people at the same time.

Excavation: the act of removing earth that is covering very old objects buried in the ground in order to discover things about the past.

Excision: the act of removing tissue, organs, or tumours in an operation.

Excision arthroplasty: removal of the affected parts of the joint.

Fretting: relative low amplitude movement (oscillation and sliding) between two mechanically joined parts, under load conditions.

Frontal plane: a frontal/coronal plane is any vertical plane that divides the body into ventral and dorsal sections (front and back). It is one of the three main planes of the body used to describe the location of body parts in relation to each other.

Hip arthroplasty/replacement: is a surgical procedure in which the hip joint is replaced by a prosthetic implant, that is, a hip prosthesis.

Horizontal plane: the transverse plane or axial plane (also called the horizontal plane or transverse plane) is an imaginary plane that divides the body into superior and inferior parts. It is perpendicular to the coronal plane and sagittal plane.

Implant: to put an organ, group of cells, or device into the body in a medical operation.

In vivo: implanted inside the patient's body

Joint stability: refers to the resistance offered by various musculoskeletal tissues that surround a skeletal joint.

Kinematics: the branch of mechanics concerned with the motion of objects without reference to the forces which cause the motion.

Knee arthroplasty: also known as knee replacement, is a surgical procedure to replace the weight-bearing surfaces of the knee joint to relieve pain and disability.

Knee replacement: also known as knee arthroplasty, is a surgical procedure to replace the weight-bearing surfaces of the knee joint to relieve pain and disability.

Lateral: relating to the sides of an object or plant or to sideways movement.

Life expectancy: the length of time that a living thing, especially a human being, is likely to live.

Ligament: any of the strong fibres (= strips of tissue) in the body that connect bones together, limiting movements in joints and supporting muscles and other tissue.

Material Specifications: A document which completely describes the fibre material used in the rope, including the material chemical composition, the fibre producer, etc.

Medial: towards the centre of the body rather than the sides.

Metres per second is an SI derived unit of both speed (scalar quantity) and velocity (vector quantity which have direction and magnitude), equal to the speed of a body covering a distance of one metre in a time of one second.

Osseointegration: is the direct structural and functional connection between living bone and the surface of a load-bearing artificial implant.

Osteolysis: bone resorption due to biological response to debris including osteoclast activation that can compromise the bone stock around the implant and lead to loosening of the prosthesis in the advanced phase.

Pre/Post-op: "Pre-op" refers to the time immediately before the day of the surgery, and "post-op" means post-operative or after surgery.

Proximal: near to the centre of the body or to the point of attachment of a bone or muscle.

Opposite: distal (away from a particular point in the body).

Resurfacing surgery: Hip (or knee) resurfacing is a type of hip replacement which replaces the surfaces of the hip joint. The procedure preserves more bone than a total hip replacement.

Rheumatism: a medical condition that causes stiffness and pain in the joints or muscles of the body.

Rheumatoid arthritis: a disease that causes stiffness, swelling, and pain in the joints of the body.

Risk factor: something that increases a person's chances of developing a disease. For example, cigarette smoking is a risk factor for lung cancer.

ROM: joint range of motion refers to both the distance a joint can move and the direction in which it can move. There are established ranges that doctors consider normal for various joints in the body.

Sagittal plane: a sagittal plane, or longitudinal plane, is an anatomical plane which divides the body into right and left parts. The plane may be in the centre of the body and split it into two halves or away from the midline and split it into unequal parts.

Soft tissue: refers to tissues that connect, support, or surround other structures and organs of the body.

Sport related injury: Sports injuries are injuries that occur when engaging in sports or exercise. Sports injuries can occur due to overtraining, lack of conditioning, and improper form or technique.

Stability: the state of being firmly fixed or not likely to move or change.

Subluxation: the partial dislocation or incomplete separation of the prosthetic joint components.

Surgical technique: the art, practice, or work of treating diseases, injuries, or deformities by manual or operative procedures.

Tegner activity scale: a one-item score that graded activity based on work and sports activities on a scale of 0 to 10. Zero represents disability because of knee/hip problems and 10 represents national or international level soccer.

Tendon: a strong piece of tissue in the body connecting a muscle to a bone.

Tissue: a group of connected cells in an animal or plant that are similar to each other, have the same purpose, and form the stated part of the animal or plan.

Tribology: the science that studies friction, lubrication and wear between two surfaces which are in close contact and move one on the other.

The name is derived from the Greek word "Τριβος," which means rubbing.

Trochlear Groove: The trochlear groove is the concave surface where the patella (kneecap) makes contact with the femur (thighbone).

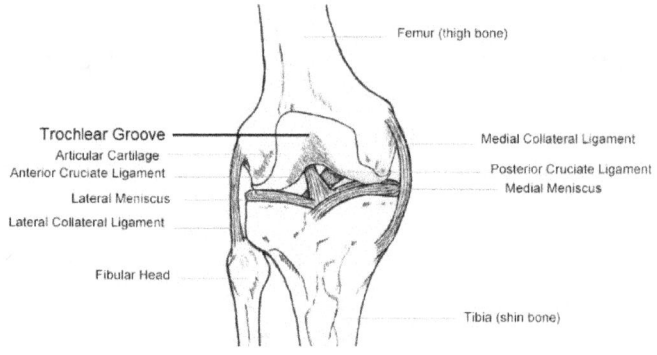

UHMWPE (ultra high molecular weight polyethylene): For over 40 years, UHMWPE has been the chosen material to use within the production of medical implant applications. Ultra-high-molecular-weight polyethylene, otherwise known as UHMWPE, has been relied upon due to its high resistance to abrasion and wear, including its incredibly strong and durable properties. There is also a newer generation PE available on the market called "HXLPE" or highly cross-linked polyethylene.

Uncemented: Bone cement was not used for implant fixation.

Wear: the surface damage with progressive loss of material (debris) due to friction between moving surfaces.

Appendix 2 - Gold/Brass Coloured Components

TiN, or titanium nitride, is a coating material that is sometimes applied to the surfaces of hip and knee implants. TiN coating has specific advantages and is used for several reasons:

Enhanced Wear Resistance: TiN is extremely hard and has excellent wear resistance properties. When applied as a coating to the metal surfaces of joint implants, it helps reduce friction and wear between the moving parts of the implant. This can extend the lifespan of the implant and reduce the likelihood of premature failure.

Improved Biocompatibility: Titanium nitride is generally biocompatible, which means it is well-tolerated by the human body. When applied as a coating, it does not typically cause adverse reactions or allergies in patients.

Reduced Metal Ion Release: By reducing wear and friction on the implant's surface, TiN coatings can help minimise the release of metal ions into the surrounding tissues. This is important because the release of metal ions can lead to adverse reactions or complications in some patients.

Improved Biomechanical Properties: TiN coatings may improve the biomechanical properties of the implant surface, making it smoother and more resistant to scratching and damage.

Enhanced Bonding: TiN coatings can enhance the bond between the implant material (often titanium or a titanium alloy) and bone. This can promote better osseointegration, where the patient's natural bone grows and bonds with the implant for added stability.

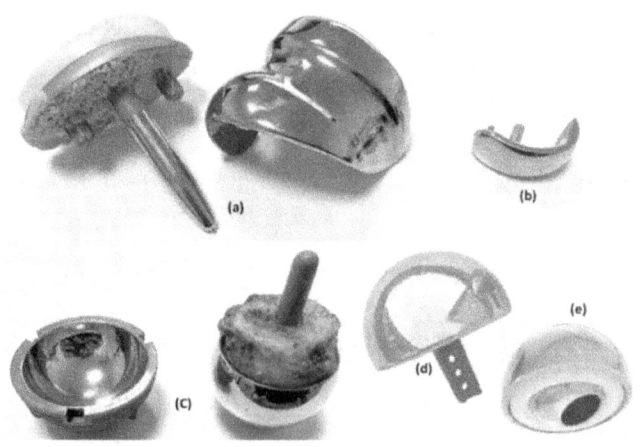

Examples of different TiN coated implants; (a) TKR, (b) UKR, (c) hip resurfacing, (d) shoulder replacement, and (e) a dual-mobility hip (by The Royal National Orthopaedic Hospital)

Appendix 3 – BMI or Body Mass Index

As explained in section I of this book, obesity (checking patient's weight and/or body mass index) is an important risk factor for a successful hip and/or knee replacement.

World Health Organisation (WHO), defines BMI as a measure for indicating nutritional status in adults. It is defined as a person's weight in kilograms divided by the square of the person's height in metres (kg/m2).

For example, an adult who weighs 70 kg and whose height is 1.75 m will have a BMI of 22.9.

$$70 \ (kg)/1.75^2 \ (m^2) = 22.9 \ BMI$$

In the USA, there have been reports that surgeons do not agree to perform joint replacement surgery on "obesity class II and III" patients. It is believed that, the hospital and insurance guidelines drive this restriction. However, this is not a universal rule & even in the US there are surgeons who perform hip and/or knee replacement on all patients

BMI classifications table by the United Nations:

BMI	Status
Below 18.5	Underweight
18.5–24.9	Normal weight
25.0–29.9	Pre-obesity
30.0–34.9	Obesity class I
35.0–39.9	Obesity class II
Above 40	Obesity class III

Having said that, critics argue BMI isn't perfect because it doesn't consider body composition and genetic differences when identifying whether someone is healthy or obese. One big issue is that BMI doesn't distinguish between types of fat and where they are in the body. For example, having excess fat around the abdomen, known as abdominal obesity, is linked to various health problems, including type 2 diabetes.

Genetics also play a role in how fat is distributed. Some Indians with a specific gene mutation (THSD7A) tend to store more fat in the abdomen, increasing the risk of health issues related to abdominal obesity, even if their overall BMI seems normal. This shows the need for a more detailed way of assessing health beyond just BMI.

BMI doesn't account for important factors like age, gender, and the balance between muscle and fat. The same BMI might mean different things for a young, muscular person compared to an older individual with more body fat. It also overlooks the difference between subcutaneous fat (under the skin) and visceral fat (around internal organs), with visceral fat posing a higher health risk.

Moreover, comparing BMI across different populations, for example Indians and Americans, doesn't make sense due to structural and genetic variations. A BMI of 25 in someone from India doesn't carry the same health implications as the same BMI in an American. Recognising these flaws in BMI calls for a reevaluation, emphasising the need for more personalised assessments to truly understand an individual's health status.

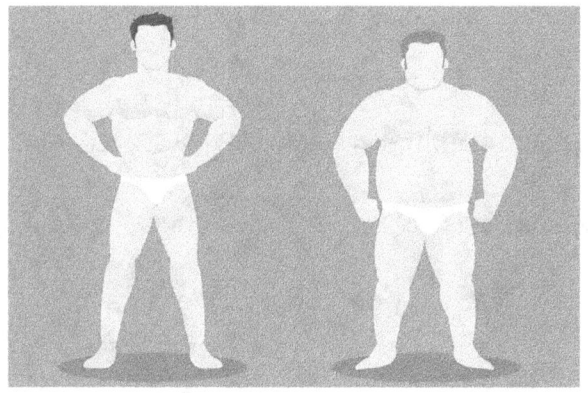

Both of these individuals share a BMI of 25.4 (pre-obesity). However, the person on the left is taller at 185cm with a muscular build. On the right, the person is shorter at 175cm & weighs 78kg, appearing to have a chubbier physique.

Appendix 4 – Pre-Surgery Preparation Checklist

Improving your general health! Depending on where you are on waiting list, you may have a couple of weeks/months to prepare by:

☐ Remaining physically active as much as you can just by making small changes e.g. if you cannot walk to work or your local supermarket, drive there but park your car further from your destination than you would normally do. This would give you the opportunity to walk.

☐ Re-evaluate your eating habits and the type of food that you eat. Avoid fast food and remember that a well-nourished body would heal more efficiently, and your recovery may be positively affected by this.

☐ Check with your doctor whether you would need to add calcium, iron or any other vitamin supplements to your diet and how much. Taking vitamins without consulting with your doctor can be dangerous.

☐ Your level of activity will naturally decrease a couple of days prior to your operation, during the operation and a few days after the operation. Besides that, some of the medication you would be given (oral or injection) during that period could cause constipation. It is important that you increase fibre and liquid intake prior to your surgery to tackle this problem.

☐ Think a head of the time and plan for the day of the surgery and a few days (to a week or two) after surgery.

☐ Arrange for someone (a family member or a friend) to accompany you on the day of your surgery.

☐ If you live by yourself, ask a family member or a friend to come to your house and stay with you for a few days after the surgery. It is likely that you will not be able to run the house the way you would normally do in the first few days after your operation until you get a little more comfortable with your new joint replacement.

☐ If you live by yourself, you would need someone "on call" for at least a couple of weeks after the surgery, so you can contact them if and when you need assistance around the house or if you need help with food shopping or taking the pet to the vet, etc.

☐ Declutter your house, remove common safety hazards and make a safe environment ready for your return from the hospital. After the surgery, you will not be able to stretch out or bend down, everything you need inside or outside of your house must be positioned in reach.

Chapter 5 - Appendices

☐ Stairs or steps outside and inside of the house must be clutter-free and it is recommended to install rails on both sides of your stairs if possible and make sure there are no slipping or falling hazards.

☐ Loose carpets or rugs, cables and wires on the floor or anything that may cause a trip or fall hazard must be removed and put away.

☐ Declutter your kitchen worktops and cabinets and make sure not to put anything inside the high wall cabinets as you must not stretch out and reach for your cereal box for example from the cabinet on top of the fridge.

☐ When walking around the house take your time, be careful and always watch out for your pets.

☐ Make sure all areas that you are likely to be walking in at night are well lit. Installing sensor lights are recommended if you are used to waking up at night to go to the bathroom, kitchen or any other room.

☐ Remember for the first few days after the operation, you will be walking with either a walker or two crutches. So, if you are used to carrying your mobile phone or a glass of water around the house with you, then make/buy a small mobile holder with a strap or a reusable bottle with a finger or wrist strap to be able to carry them around the house whilst walking with your crutches.

☐ Take a good look at your bathroom, take some time and see how you can improve your bathroom environment to a safer area. Some suggestions are decluttering, changing your bath mat with a non-slip mat, installing shower rails, buying a raised toilet seat and definitely keep your toilet paper at reach especially if you have had a hip replacement as picking up toilet roll (or your pants) off of the bathroom floor whilst sat on the toilet seat is a common reason for hip dislocation.

Notes..

Notes

Notes

www.ingramcontent.com/pod-product-compliance
Lightning Source LLC
Chambersburg PA
CBHW071348210526
45465CB00001B/21